SKINCARE SOLUTIONS: EFFECTIVE TREATMENTS FOR EVERY SKIN TYPE

How to Tackle Acne, Aging, and Other Skin Issues with Targeted Treatments and Practical Advice

GENNIFER RED

INTRODUCTION: THE SKINCARE REVOLUTION

Overview of Modern Skincare

In recent years, skincare has evolved from a basic routine of cleansing and moisturizing into a sophisticated practice that is deeply rooted in science. Modern skincare is no longer just about maintaining a clean and hydrated complexion; it is a comprehensive approach to understanding and treating the skin at a cellular level. This shift reflects a growing awareness of the intricate relationship between skin health and overall well-being.

At the heart of this revolution is the increased focus on the science behind skincare products and treatments. Gone are the days when consumers were satisfied with vague promises of "radiant" or "glowing" skin. Today, people want to know exactly how a product works, what ingredients it contains, and what benefits it can offer. This demand for transparency and efficacy has pushed the skincare industry to prioritize research and development, leading to the creation of highly specialized products designed to address specific skin concerns.

One of the main challenges in modern skincare is the sheer variety of products and ingredients available on the market. With thousands of serums, creams, and treatments to choose from, it can be overwhelming for consumers to determine what is best for their skin type. This is where the importance of personalized skincare comes into play. Rather than following a one-size-fits-all approach, modern skincare emphasizes the need for routines that are tailored to individual needs. Understanding your skin type, identifying specific concerns like acne, aging, or hyperpigmentation, and selecting products that target these issues are crucial steps in developing an effective skincare regimen.

Another significant aspect of modern skincare is the growing recognition of the impact of external factors on skin health. Environmental aggressors such as pollution, UV radiation, and even stress can exacerbate skin issues and accelerate the aging process. As a result, many contemporary skincare products are formulated with ingredients that protect the skin from these external threats while simultaneously addressing internal factors like hormonal changes and diet. This holistic approach underscores the complexity of skin health and the need for comprehensive care that goes beyond surface-level treatment.

In addition to the scientific advancements in skincare, there is also a cultural shift towards self-care and wellness. Skincare routines are increasingly seen as a form of self-expression and self-care, offering individuals a moment of calm and control in their daily lives. This perspective not only enhances the emotional and psychological benefits of skincare but also encourages a deeper commitment to maintaining skin health over the long term.

As we delve into the various aspects of skincare throughout this book, it is essential to recognize that the true revolution in skincare lies in this blend of science, personalization, and self-care. By understanding the principles of modern skincare and applying them thoughtfully, you can achieve not just healthier skin, but a more informed and empowered approach to your overall well-being.

Why This Book?

In the vast and ever-expanding world of skincare, finding reliable, scientifically-backed information can be a daunting task. With countless products on the market, each promising miraculous results, and a plethora of advice available online, it's easy to feel overwhelmed and uncertain about what truly works. This book was created to cut through the noise and provide you with a clear, practical guide to taking care of your skin effectively.

The value of this book lies in its foundation on both scientific research and practical application. Unlike many sources that offer superficial advice or promote the latest trends without substantiation, this book is rooted in a deep understanding of dermatology and skin biology. Each chapter is designed to educate you on the principles of skincare, from understanding your skin's unique needs to selecting the right products and treatments. This approach ensures that you are not just following routines blindly but are empowered with knowledge that allows you to make informed decisions about your skincare.

One of the key reasons this book is essential is its focus on personalization. Skin is a complex organ that varies significantly from person to person, influenced by factors such as genetics, environment, age, and lifestyle. What works for one individual may not work for another. This book acknowledges that diversity and provides tailored advice to address a wide range of skin types and concerns. Whether you are dealing with acne, aging, sensitivity, or hyperpigmentation, you will find specific strategies and recommendations that cater to your particular needs.

Another significant aspect of this book is its commitment to demystifying the science behind skincare. In an industry often shrouded in marketing jargon and pseudoscience, it can be challenging to differentiate between what is truly effective and what is mere hype. This book breaks down complex scientific concepts into understandable language, explaining how various ingredients and treatments work at a cellular level. This knowledge not only helps you choose products more wisely but also gives you confidence in your skincare decisions.

Practicality is at the heart of this book's mission. While understanding the science is crucial, it's equally important that you can apply this knowledge in a way that fits into your daily life. The advice and routines outlined in this book are designed to be realistic and sustainable. We recognize that modern life is busy, and not everyone has the time or resources to follow an elaborate skincare regimen. Therefore, the guidance provided is straightforward and actionable, allowing you to integrate effective skincare practices into your routine without feeling overwhelmed.

Lastly, this book serves as a reliable resource in an era where misinformation is rampant. In a market saturated with conflicting advice, having a trustworthy source of information is invaluable. This book has been meticulously researched and carefully curated to ensure that every piece of advice is supported by evidence and expert consensus. By reading this book, you are equipping yourself with the tools and knowledge necessary to achieve healthier, more radiant skin, while avoiding the pitfalls of fads and misinformation.

How to Use This Book

This book is designed to be a comprehensive guide that you can return to time and again as you navigate your skincare journey. Whether you are just beginning to explore the world of skincare or are looking to refine your existing routine, this book provides the tools and knowledge you need to achieve your skin goals. Understanding how to effectively use this book will help you tailor its contents to your specific needs, ensuring that you get the most out of every chapter.

Each chapter of this book is structured to build upon the previous one, starting with the fundamentals of skin science and progressing through the intricacies of skincare ingredients, routines, and treatments. However, you don't necessarily need to read it from cover to cover in one sitting. Depending on your current level of knowledge and specific concerns, you might find it more beneficial to jump to the sections that are most relevant to you. For example, if you're primarily concerned with anti-aging, you might begin with the chapter on advanced treatments for aging skin before circling back to the basics of skincare.

To help you navigate the book, each chapter is broken down into clear, manageable sections that focus on specific topics. This structure allows you to quickly find the information you need without feeling overwhelmed. If you're dealing with a particular issue, such as acne or hyperpigmentation, you can easily locate the relevant chapter and dive into the targeted advice and strategies offered there. The table of contents and chapter summaries are designed to guide you to the right place, making it easy to access the information you need when you need it.

As you read through the book, you'll notice that it emphasizes the importance of personalization. Skincare is not a one-size-fits-all endeavor, and the advice provided in this book is meant to be adapted to your unique skin type, concerns, and lifestyle. To help you with this, each chapter includes practical tips on how to customize the general advice to suit your individual needs. For instance, when discussing skincare routines, the book offers different recommendations based on whether you have dry, oily, combination, or sensitive skin. Take the time to assess your skin's specific characteristics and use the guidelines provided to modify the suggestions accordingly.

The book also encourages you to take a proactive approach to your skincare by keeping track of your progress and adjusting your routine as needed. Skin can change over time due to factors like age, climate, and health, so it's important to remain flexible and responsive to these changes. The book includes sections that guide you on how to monitor your skin's condition, identify when adjustments are necessary, and implement those changes effectively.

To maximize the benefits of this book, consider it as both an educational resource and a practical tool. Use the knowledge you gain to make informed decisions about the products and routines you choose. Revisit the chapters as your skin changes or as new questions arise. By actively engaging with the content and applying the advice to your daily routine, you will be better equipped to achieve and maintain healthy, radiant skin.

SOMMARIO

CHAPTER 1: UNDERSTANDING THE SKIN

1.1 The Science of Skin

The human skin is a remarkable organ, not only because it is the largest in the body but also due to its complexity and the vital roles it plays in maintaining overall health. To truly understand how to care for your skin, it's essential to grasp the basics of its structure and function. The skin is composed of three primary layers: the epidermis, the dermis, and the hypodermis. Each of these layers has distinct functions that contribute to the skin's protective, sensory, and regulatory roles.

The **epidermis** is the outermost layer of the skin, acting as the first line of defense against environmental aggressors such as bacteria, viruses, and harmful UV rays. This layer is composed mainly of keratinocytes, which are cells that produce keratin, a protein that provides the skin with its toughness and water-resistant properties. The epidermis is further divided into sub-layers, including the stratum corneum, which is the outermost sub-layer and consists of dead skin cells that are continually shed and replaced. Beneath it lies the stratum granulosum, where cells begin to lose their nuclei and start the process of keratinization. The stratum spinosum and stratum basale are the deeper sub-layers, where active cell division occurs, producing new cells that eventually migrate to the surface.

Another crucial component of the epidermis is **melanocytes**, the cells responsible for producing melanin, the pigment that gives skin its color and provides some protection against UV radiation. The amount and type of melanin produced determine an individual's skin tone and how their skin reacts to sun exposure. Additionally, the epidermis contains Langerhans cells, which are part of the immune system and play a role in detecting and fighting off pathogens that may penetrate the skin.

Beneath the epidermis lies the **dermis**, a thicker layer that provides structural support and nourishment to the skin. The dermis is composed of a dense network of collagen and elastin fibers, which give the skin its strength, elasticity, and resilience. Collagen, the most abundant protein in the dermis, forms a scaffold that supports the skin and keeps it firm. Elastin fibers allow the skin to stretch and return to its original shape, which is particularly important in areas of the body that experience frequent movement.

The dermis is also home to various structures essential for skin function, including blood vessels, nerves, sweat glands, and sebaceous glands. Blood vessels in the dermis deliver oxygen and nutrients to the skin cells while also aiding in temperature regulation by widening or constricting in response to external conditions. Nerves in the dermis are responsible for the skin's sensory functions, allowing us to feel touch, pain, and temperature. Sweat glands help regulate body temperature by releasing sweat, which cools the body as it evaporates. Sebaceous glands produce sebum, an oily substance that lubricates and waterproofs the skin and hair.

The innermost layer of the skin is the **hypodermis**, also known as the subcutaneous layer. This layer is primarily composed of adipose tissue, which stores fat and provides insulation and cushioning for the body. The hypodermis also serves as an energy reserve and helps anchor the skin to underlying structures such as muscles and bones. While the hypodermis is not directly involved in the surface functions of the skin, its role in insulation and cushioning is vital for overall protection and temperature regulation.

Understanding the structure of the skin and the specific functions of each layer is crucial for making informed decisions about skincare. The health and appearance of your skin depend on how well these layers perform their roles, and skincare practices should aim to support and enhance the natural processes that occur within the skin. By recognizing the complexities of your skin, you can better appreciate the importance of using products and treatments that align with your skin's unique needs, ultimately leading to healthier and more resilient skin.

1.2 The Different Skin Types

Understanding your skin type is the foundation of an effective skincare routine. Each person's skin has unique characteristics that determine how it reacts to various products, environmental factors, and internal changes. There are four main skin types— normal, dry, oily, and combination—each with its own set of traits and challenges. Identifying your skin type is crucial in choosing the right skincare products and routines to maintain healthy, balanced skin.

Normal Skin

Normal skin is often considered the ideal skin type due to its balanced nature. It has a healthy level of moisture, sufficient oil production, and good blood circulation. People with normal skin typically have a smooth texture, small pores, and a radiant complexion. This skin type is neither too oily nor too dry, and it rarely experiences severe breakouts or irritation.

One of the defining characteristics of normal skin is its ability to maintain equilibrium even when exposed to varying environmental conditions. It can handle changes in humidity, temperature, and diet without becoming overly reactive. Normal skin also tends to recover quickly from minor skin issues, such as a pimple or dry patch, without leaving significant marks or scars.

While normal skin is generally low maintenance, it still requires regular care to preserve its balance. A basic skincare routine that includes cleansing, moisturizing, and sun protection is essential. Additionally, incorporating antioxidants and mild exfoliants can help maintain the skin's youthful appearance and prevent early signs of aging.

Dry Skin

Dry skin is characterized by a lack of natural moisture and oil, which can lead to a tight, rough, and sometimes flaky appearance. This skin type often feels uncomfortable, especially after cleansing or during cold, dry weather. The lack of oil production in dry skin means that the protective barrier is weaker, making it more prone to irritation, redness, and fine lines.

One of the key indicators of dry skin is a dull complexion. Without sufficient oil to lock in moisture, the skin can look lackluster and feel rough to the touch. Dry skin may also have visibly fine lines or cracks, particularly around the eyes and mouth, where the skin is thinner and more delicate.

To care for dry skin, it's important to focus on hydration and nourishment. Using gentle, non-foaming cleansers that do not strip the skin of its natural oils is crucial. Moisturizers rich in emollients, such as shea butter, ceramides, and hyaluronic acid, can help restore the skin's barrier and retain moisture.

Additionally, incorporating hydrating serums and oils into the routine can provide extra nourishment. Regular use of a humidifier in dry climates can also be beneficial in maintaining skin hydration.

Oily Skin

Oily skin is characterized by an overproduction of sebum, the natural oil produced by the sebaceous glands. This excess oil can lead to a shiny appearance, enlarged pores, and a greater propensity for acne and blackheads. People with oily skin often notice that their face becomes greasy throughout the day, particularly in the T-zone area (forehead, nose, and chin).

The primary advantage of oily skin is that it tends to be more resilient and less prone to fine lines and wrinkles compared to dry skin. The natural oils provide a protective barrier that helps prevent moisture loss and shields the skin from environmental aggressors. However, the downside is that the excess oil can clog pores, leading to the development of acne, blackheads, and other blemishes.

Managing oily skin involves finding the right balance between controlling oil production and maintaining adequate hydration. Foaming or gel-based cleansers that remove excess oil without over-drying the skin are ideal. Exfoliating regularly with salicylic acid or glycolic acid can help prevent clogged pores and reduce breakouts. Lightweight, non-comedogenic moisturizers that do not add extra oil but provide necessary hydration are essential. Additionally, using clay masks once or twice a week can help absorb excess oil and refine pores.

Combination Skin

Combination skin is perhaps the most common and complex skin type, as it displays characteristics of both oily and dry skin. Typically, people with combination skin experience an oily T-zone, with dryness or normal skin on the cheeks and other areas of the face. This dual nature can make it challenging to find skincare products that address both the oiliness and dryness simultaneously.

One of the telltale signs of combination skin is the contrast between the different areas of the face. The T-zone may appear shiny and prone to breakouts, while the cheeks may feel tight, dry, or even flaky. This skin type requires a customized approach to care, as treating the oily and dry areas with the same products can lead to further imbalance.

For combination skin, it's important to use different products for different areas of the face or to choose products that are designed to balance the skin's overall condition. A gentle, balancing cleanser that removes impurities without stripping the skin is a good starting point. Lightweight, hydrating moisturizers that provide moisture without clogging pores are ideal for the entire face, while spot treatments with salicylic acid can be applied to the oily areas to control breakouts. Additionally, using a hydrating serum or oil-free moisturizer on the drier areas can help maintain the skin's balance.

Identifying Your Skin Type

Determining your skin type is the first step in developing an effective skincare routine. One simple method to identify your skin type is the bare-faced test. Start by washing your face with a gentle cleanser, then pat it dry and wait for about an hour. During this time, avoid applying any skincare products. After the hour has passed, observe how your skin feels and looks.

- If your skin feels comfortable and balanced without any noticeable oiliness or dryness, you likely have normal skin.

- If your skin feels tight, rough, or flaky, particularly around the cheeks, you likely have dry skin.

- If your skin appears shiny, especially in the T-zone, and feels greasy to the touch, you likely have oily skin.

- If your T-zone is oily but your cheeks are dry or normal, you likely have combination skin.

Another method to identify your skin type is by observing how your skin reacts throughout the day. If you notice that your skin becomes greasy quickly after washing, it's a sign of oily skin. If your skin feels tight or looks dull by the end of the day, it's likely dry. For those with combination skin, the T-zone may become oily while the rest of the face remains dry or comfortable.

Understanding your skin type is crucial for selecting the right skincare products and treatments. It helps you avoid products that could exacerbate issues like dryness, oiliness, or breakouts and instead choose those that support and enhance your skin's natural balance. By identifying your skin type, you can tailor your skincare routine to meet your specific needs, leading to healthier, more radiant skin.

1.3 Factors That Influence the Skin

The condition of your skin is the result of a complex interplay between internal and external factors. Understanding these influences is key to managing your skin's health and appearance effectively. Internal factors such as genetics, hormones, and age are intrinsic and largely out of your control, while external factors like climate, pollution, and stress can be managed to some extent through lifestyle choices and skincare practices. Each of these factors plays a significant role in how your skin looks and feels, and recognizing their effects can help you tailor your skincare routine to address specific needs.

Internal Factors

Genetics

Genetics is one of the most fundamental internal factors influencing your skin type, texture, and overall condition. Your genetic makeup determines how your skin responds to various stimuli, including environmental factors, aging, and hormonal changes. For instance, genetics play a significant role in the natural oil production of your skin, which in turn influences whether your skin is dry, oily, or somewhere in between. Additionally, genetic predispositions can affect your skin's sensitivity, its likelihood to develop certain conditions such as acne or rosacea, and even how it heals from wounds or blemishes.

While you cannot change your genetic makeup, understanding its impact on your skin can guide you in choosing the right skincare products and treatments. For example, if you have a family history of acne or eczema, you might be more vigilant in managing these conditions through targeted skincare and lifestyle choices. Similarly, if your genetics predispose you to early signs of aging, such as fine lines or loss of elasticity, you can focus on preventive measures like using sunscreen, antioxidants, and collagen-boosting ingredients from a younger age.

Hormones

Hormones are another critical internal factor that significantly affects your skin's condition. Hormonal fluctuations occur naturally throughout life, influenced by puberty, menstruation, pregnancy, and menopause. These fluctuations can cause various skin changes, such as increased oil production leading to acne, or a decrease in collagen production resulting in wrinkles and sagging skin.

During puberty, the surge in androgens (male hormones present in both sexes) stimulates the sebaceous glands to produce more oil, which can clog pores and lead to acne. Similarly, hormonal changes during pregnancy can cause hyperpigmentation, often referred to as "pregnancy mask" or melasma, due to increased levels of estrogen and progesterone.

Menopause brings about a significant decline in estrogen levels, which can lead to thinner, drier skin and the acceleration of aging signs. Understanding these hormonal effects is crucial for adjusting your skincare routine accordingly. For instance, during periods of hormonal fluctuations, incorporating products that regulate oil production, boost hydration, or target hyperpigmentation can help maintain skin balance and reduce the risk of skin issues.

Age

Aging is an inevitable internal factor that profoundly impacts the skin over time. As we age, the skin's ability to regenerate and repair itself diminishes. The production of collagen and elastin, the proteins responsible for skin's firmness and elasticity, decreases, leading to sagging skin, fine lines, and wrinkles. Additionally, the skin's natural exfoliation process slows down, resulting in a buildup of dead skin cells that can cause a dull, uneven complexion.

Another age-related change is the reduction in sebum production, which can lead to drier skin as you get older. This decline in oil production, combined with the thinning of the skin's outer layer, makes the skin more susceptible to damage from environmental factors like UV rays and pollution.

To address the effects of aging, it's important to adapt your skincare routine over time. Incorporating products that stimulate collagen production, such as retinoids and peptides, can help maintain skin firmness. Using moisturizers with hyaluronic acid and ceramides can combat dryness, while regular exfoliation with gentle acids can keep the skin looking bright and smooth.

External Factors

Climate

Climate is one of the most influential external factors affecting your skin. Depending on where you live, the weather can have a variety of effects on your skin's condition. For instance, cold, dry climates can strip the skin of its natural moisture, leading to dryness, flakiness, and irritation. In contrast, hot and humid climates can increase sweat and oil production, making the skin more prone to breakouts and shine.

Seasonal changes also play a role in how your skin behaves. During the winter, lower humidity levels can dehydrate the skin, making it necessary to use richer moisturizers and possibly increase the use of hydrating serums. Conversely, in the summer, the combination of heat and humidity may require lighter skincare products and increased use of sunscreen to protect against UV rays.

Tailoring your skincare routine to the climate is essential for maintaining healthy skin year-round. This might include switching to different types of cleansers, moisturizers, and sunscreens depending on the season or your geographical location.

Pollution

Pollution, particularly in urban environments, is a significant external factor that can have detrimental effects on the skin. Airborne pollutants such as smog, dust, and chemical particles can settle on the skin, leading to clogged pores, irritation, and the breakdown of collagen and elastin. Over time, exposure to pollution can accelerate the aging process, resulting in premature wrinkles, uneven skin tone, and loss of elasticity.

Pollution also contributes to oxidative stress, which occurs when the skin is exposed to free radicals—unstable molecules that damage cells and DNA. This oxidative stress can weaken the skin's barrier function, making it more susceptible to damage and inflammation.

To protect your skin from pollution, it's important to incorporate antioxidants into your skincare routine. Ingredients like vitamin C, vitamin E, and green tea extract can neutralize free radicals and help prevent damage. Additionally, thoroughly cleansing your skin at the end of the day to remove pollutants is crucial, and using products that strengthen the skin's barrier, such as niacinamide, can help defend against environmental aggressors.

Stress

Stress is an often-overlooked external factor that can have a profound impact on your skin. When you are stressed, your body produces higher levels of cortisol, a hormone that can trigger increased oil production, leading to acne and other skin issues. Chronic stress can also disrupt the skin's barrier function, making it more prone to sensitivity, redness, and irritation.

Stress can exacerbate existing skin conditions like eczema, psoriasis, and rosacea, causing flare-ups and making these conditions more difficult to manage. Additionally, stress can interfere with your sleep patterns, which in turn affects skin regeneration and repair, leading to a tired, dull complexion.

Managing stress is essential for maintaining healthy skin. Incorporating stress-reducing activities such as exercise, meditation, and adequate sleep can improve both your overall well-being and your skin's condition. Additionally, using soothing skincare products that contain ingredients like chamomile, aloe vera, and lavender can help calm stressed skin and reduce inflammation.

Lifestyle Choices

Beyond the specific factors mentioned, various lifestyle choices also play a role in your skin's health. Diet, hydration, sleep, and exercise all contribute to how your skin looks and feels. A diet rich in vitamins, minerals, and antioxidants can provide the nutrients your skin needs to repair and regenerate. Drinking plenty of water helps keep your skin hydrated from the inside out, while regular exercise improves circulation, bringing more oxygen and nutrients to the skin.

Sleep is particularly important for skin health, as it is during sleep that the body repairs and regenerates cells. Lack of sleep can lead to dark circles, puffiness, and a dull complexion. Prioritizing sleep and maintaining a balanced diet and exercise routine are simple yet effective ways to support your skin's overall health.

By understanding the various internal and external factors that influence your skin, you can take a more holistic approach to skincare. This means not only selecting the right products but also making lifestyle adjustments that support your skin's health from the inside out. Through a combination of targeted skincare and healthy habits, you can better manage the impact of these factors and achieve a more radiant, resilient complexion.

1.4 Common Skin Issues

Skin issues are a universal concern, affecting people of all ages, skin types, and backgrounds. Understanding these common problems is the first step in addressing them effectively. This section introduces some of the most prevalent skin conditions—acne, rosacea, sensitivity, and aging—and explores how they manifest differently across various skin types.

Acne

Acne is one of the most common skin conditions, affecting millions of people worldwide. It occurs when hair follicles become clogged with oil and dead skin cells, leading to the formation of pimples, blackheads, and whiteheads. Acne is most commonly associated with oily skin, where excess sebum production contributes to the clogging of pores. However, it can also affect those with combination or even dry skin, especially in areas prone to higher oil production, like the T-zone.

Hormonal fluctuations, particularly during puberty, menstruation, and pregnancy, can exacerbate acne by increasing oil production. Stress, diet, and the use of pore-clogging skincare products can also contribute to breakouts. Acne manifests as red, inflamed pimples or cysts, and in severe cases, it can lead to scarring. For those with oily skin, acne is often persistent, requiring careful management with products that balance oil production and keep pores clear. Those with combination skin may experience breakouts primarily in the T-zone, while individuals with dry skin might see occasional acne due to environmental factors or incorrect product use.

Rosacea

Rosacea is a chronic skin condition that causes redness, visible blood vessels, and sometimes acne-like bumps on the face. It typically affects those with fair skin, but it can occur in any skin type. The exact cause of rosacea is unknown, but it is believed to be related to a combination of genetic and environmental factors, such as sun exposure, heat, spicy foods, and stress.

Rosacea is more common in adults over 30 and often presents as persistent redness on the cheeks, nose, forehead, and chin. In more severe cases, it can cause the skin to thicken and swell, particularly around the nose, a condition known as rhinophyma. People with rosacea often have sensitive skin that is easily irritated by skincare products and environmental factors. Managing rosacea involves avoiding known triggers, using gentle skincare products, and sometimes seeking medical treatment to control symptoms. Individuals with combination skin may notice that the oily areas of their face are more prone to rosacea flare-ups, while those with dry skin might experience more irritation and dryness as a result of the condition.

Skin Sensitivity

Skin sensitivity is characterized by a heightened reaction to external factors, such as skincare products, environmental changes, and even stress. Sensitive skin often reacts with redness, itching, burning, or dryness, making it challenging to find suitable skincare products that do not cause irritation. Sensitivity can occur in any skin type but is more common in dry and combination skin, where the skin's barrier is compromised or more prone to reactions.

Several factors contribute to skin sensitivity, including genetics, environmental exposure, and the overuse of harsh skincare products. People with sensitive skin may experience flare-ups in response to common irritants such as fragrances, alcohol-based products, and certain preservatives. Sensitivity can also be aggravated by environmental conditions like cold weather, wind, and pollution, which further compromise the skin's protective barrier.

To manage sensitive skin, it's crucial to focus on strengthening the skin's barrier with gentle, hydrating products that are free from common irritants. Ingredients like ceramides, hyaluronic acid, and niacinamide can help soothe and protect sensitive skin, while avoiding known triggers is essential for minimizing flare-ups.

Aging

Aging is a natural process that affects the skin's appearance and function over time. As we age, the skin undergoes several changes, including a decrease in collagen and elastin production, which leads to the development of fine lines, wrinkles, and sagging. The skin also becomes thinner, drier, and more prone to damage from environmental factors such as UV radiation and pollution.

Aging affects all skin types, but the way it manifests can vary. For example, those with dry skin may notice signs of aging earlier due to the lack of moisture, which can exacerbate the appearance of fine lines and wrinkles. In contrast, individuals with oily skin may experience delayed signs of aging, as the excess oil helps to keep the skin more hydrated and protected. However, oily skin types are not immune to aging; they may still develop wrinkles, particularly around the eyes and mouth, where the skin is thinner and more prone to movement.

Preventing and managing the signs of aging involves a combination of protective measures and targeted treatments. Sunscreen is essential for preventing UV-induced damage, while antioxidants like vitamin C and retinoids can help combat oxidative stress and stimulate collagen production. Hydration is also crucial, as well-moisturized skin is more resilient and better able to repair itself. For those with aging concerns, a tailored skincare routine that addresses specific needs, such as dryness, fine lines, and loss of elasticity, can help maintain a youthful appearance for longer.

Understanding these common skin issues and how they affect different skin types is vital for developing an effective skincare routine. By recognizing the signs and triggers of acne, rosacea, sensitivity, and aging, you can choose products and treatments that address your unique skin concerns, leading to healthier, more balanced skin.

CHAPTER 2: THE SCIENCE BEHIND INGREDIENTS

2.1 Introduction to Active Ingredients

Active ingredients are the powerhouse components of any effective skincare product. Unlike inactive ingredients, which primarily serve to deliver and stabilize the formula, active ingredients are specifically included for their therapeutic effects on the skin. These ingredients target particular skin concerns, such as aging, acne, hyperpigmentation, or hydration, and work at the cellular level to bring about noticeable changes. Understanding the role of active ingredients in skincare is crucial for selecting the right products and creating a routine that addresses your unique skin needs.

Active ingredients are what differentiate a basic moisturizer from a targeted treatment. They are the reason why certain products can smooth wrinkles, fade dark spots, or reduce acne. The effectiveness of a skincare product largely depends on the type and concentration of its active ingredients, as well as how these ingredients interact with the skin.

One of the most well-known and widely used active ingredients is **retinol**, a derivative of vitamin A. Retinol is celebrated for its ability to accelerate cell turnover, which helps to reduce the appearance of fine lines, wrinkles, and hyperpigmentation. By promoting the shedding of old, damaged skin cells and encouraging the production of new ones, retinol helps to improve skin texture and tone over time. It also stimulates collagen production, which is essential for maintaining skin firmness and elasticity. Due to its potency, retinol is often introduced gradually into a skincare routine to allow the skin to build tolerance and minimize irritation.

Vitamin C is another powerful active ingredient, known for its antioxidant properties. As an antioxidant, vitamin C neutralizes free radicals—unstable molecules that can damage skin cells and accelerate aging. Additionally, vitamin C plays a crucial role in collagen synthesis, helping to maintain skin's structural integrity and reduce the appearance of fine lines. It also has brightening properties, making it effective in treating hyperpigmentation and evening out skin tone. When formulated correctly, vitamin C can enhance the skin's natural defense mechanisms and provide a radiant, youthful glow.

Hyaluronic acid is a hydrating powerhouse that naturally occurs in the skin but decreases with age. It has the unique ability to hold up to 1,000 times its weight in water, making it incredibly effective at attracting and retaining moisture. This makes hyaluronic acid an essential ingredient for anyone looking to boost skin hydration, plump fine lines, and improve overall skin texture. Unlike some active ingredients that can be irritating, hyaluronic acid is gentle and suitable for all skin types, making it a versatile component in both moisturizers and serums.

Salicylic acid is a beta hydroxy acid (BHA) that is particularly effective for treating acne. It works by penetrating the pores and exfoliating from within, helping to remove dead skin cells and reduce oil buildup that can lead to breakouts. Salicylic acid is also anti-inflammatory, making it effective in reducing the redness and swelling associated with acne. Regular use of products containing salicylic acid can help to keep pores clear and prevent future breakouts, making it a staple in the skincare routines of those with oily or acne-prone skin.

Another important active ingredient is **niacinamide**, a form of vitamin B3 that offers multiple benefits for the skin. Niacinamide is known for its ability to improve the skin's barrier function, which helps to retain moisture and protect against environmental damage. It also has anti-inflammatory properties, making it beneficial for reducing redness and irritation. Furthermore, niacinamide can regulate oil production, minimize the appearance of pores, and even out skin tone, making it a highly versatile ingredient suitable for a range of skin concerns.

Peptides are short chains of amino acids that serve as the building blocks of proteins like collagen and elastin in the skin. As we age, the production of these proteins decreases, leading to wrinkles and loss of firmness. Peptides in skincare products can signal the skin to produce more collagen and elastin, helping to strengthen the skin's structure and reduce the signs of aging. Due to their ability to support the skin's natural processes, peptides are often included in anti-aging formulations designed to improve skin elasticity and smooth fine lines.

Alpha hydroxy acids (AHAs), such as glycolic acid and lactic acid, are another category of active ingredients that are widely used for their exfoliating properties. AHAs work by loosening the bonds between dead skin cells, allowing them to be easily removed and revealing fresher, more radiant skin underneath. Regular use of AHAs can help to improve skin texture, reduce the appearance of fine lines, and fade hyperpigmentation. However, because AHAs can increase the skin's sensitivity to the sun, it's important to use them in conjunction with a broad-spectrum sunscreen.

Ceramides are lipids (fats) that naturally occur in the skin's outer layer and are essential for maintaining the skin's barrier function. A healthy skin barrier protects against environmental aggressors, retains moisture, and prevents irritants from penetrating the skin. When the skin's ceramide levels are low, the barrier can become compromised, leading to dryness, irritation, and increased sensitivity. Skincare products containing ceramides help to replenish these lipids, restoring the skin's barrier and improving overall hydration.

The effectiveness of active ingredients is not only dependent on their presence in a product but also on their concentration and formulation. For instance, a product with a high concentration of an active ingredient like retinol or vitamin C may be more effective but also more likely to cause irritation if not used correctly. Similarly, the pH level of a product can affect the stability and absorption of active ingredients, influencing their overall efficacy.

When incorporating active ingredients into your skincare routine, it's important to consider how they work together. Some ingredients, like retinol and AHAs, can be potent and may cause irritation if used simultaneously, especially for those with sensitive skin. On the other hand, some ingredients, such as vitamin C and ferulic acid, can complement each other, enhancing their antioxidant effects and stability.

Active ingredients are the key components that give skincare products their ability to address specific concerns and improve skin health. By understanding how these ingredients work and choosing products that contain the right actives for your skin type and concerns, you can create a skincare routine that delivers real, visible results.

2.2 Peptides and the Fight Against Aging

Peptides have become a cornerstone in the fight against aging, gaining significant attention for their ability to enhance skin health and appearance at a cellular level. As short chains of amino acids, peptides serve as the building blocks of proteins, such as collagen and elastin, which are essential for maintaining the skin's structure and elasticity. As we age, the natural production of these proteins diminishes, leading to the visible signs of aging, such as wrinkles, sagging, and loss of firmness. Peptides in skincare play a crucial role in stimulating the production of these proteins, thereby helping to combat and even reverse some of the effects of aging.

One of the primary roles of peptides in skincare is to signal the skin to produce more collagen. Collagen is the most abundant protein in the skin, providing structural support and strength. However, starting in our mid-20s, the body's collagen production begins to slow down, and by the time we reach our 40s and 50s, the skin's collagen levels have significantly declined. This reduction in collagen leads to the formation of wrinkles, fine lines, and a general loss of skin elasticity and firmness.

Peptides work by mimicking the body's natural communication mechanisms. When collagen breaks down, it releases specific peptides that signal the skin to produce more collagen. By applying peptides topically, you can trick the skin into thinking that more collagen is needed, thereby stimulating collagen production. This increase in collagen helps to smooth out wrinkles, improve skin texture, and restore a youthful firmness to the skin.

There are several types of peptides used in skincare, each with its unique function and benefits. **Signal peptides**, as the name suggests, send signals to the skin to boost collagen production. These peptides are particularly effective in reducing the appearance of fine lines and wrinkles, as they directly encourage the skin to regenerate and repair itself. **Carrier peptides** deliver trace elements such as copper and magnesium to the skin, which are essential for wound healing and collagen synthesis. Copper peptides, in particular, are known for their ability to promote the production of glycosaminoglycans, like hyaluronic acid, which help maintain skin hydration and plumpness.

Enzyme-inhibiting peptides work by inhibiting the enzymes that break down collagen in the skin. By preventing this breakdown, these peptides help to preserve the skin's existing collagen, keeping it firmer and more elastic. Matrixyl, a well-known enzyme-inhibiting peptide, has been extensively studied and shown to reduce wrinkle depth and improve overall skin tone. **Neurotransmitter-inhibiting peptides** act similarly to Botox, as they reduce the contraction of facial muscles, thereby preventing the formation of dynamic wrinkles. These peptides work by blocking the release of acetylcholine, a neurotransmitter that triggers muscle contractions, leading to a temporary smoothing of expression lines.

When incorporated into a skincare routine, peptides offer several anti-aging benefits. They help to improve skin barrier function, enhance moisture retention, and promote a smoother, more even skin tone. The skin barrier is the outermost layer of the skin, responsible for protecting against environmental aggressors and retaining moisture. As we age, the skin barrier can become compromised, leading to dryness, irritation, and increased sensitivity. Peptides help to strengthen the skin barrier, making it more resilient and better able to retain moisture, which is crucial for maintaining a youthful appearance.

Peptides are also known for their ability to enhance the skin's overall texture and tone. By stimulating collagen production and inhibiting its breakdown, peptides help to reduce the appearance of fine lines and wrinkles, resulting in smoother, firmer skin. Additionally, peptides can help to even out skin tone by reducing the appearance of hyperpigmentation and promoting a more uniform complexion. This is particularly beneficial for those dealing with age spots or uneven skin tone, which are common signs of aging.

To maximize the effectiveness of peptides in skincare, it's important to use them in combination with other active ingredients that complement their action. For example, pairing peptides with antioxidants like vitamin C can help to protect the skin from free radical damage while boosting collagen production. Similarly, using peptides alongside hyaluronic acid can enhance moisture retention and plump the skin, further reducing the appearance of fine lines and wrinkles.

The formulation of peptide-containing products is also crucial for their effectiveness. Peptides are relatively small molecules, which allows them to penetrate the skin's outer layer and reach the deeper layers where collagen production occurs. However, the stability and delivery of peptides in skincare products can vary, depending on the formulation. Look for products that are designed to stabilize peptides and enhance their penetration into the skin, such as serums and creams that use encapsulation technology or other advanced delivery systems.

While peptides are generally well-tolerated by most skin types, it's important to introduce them gradually into your skincare routine, especially if you have sensitive skin. Start with a product that contains a lower concentration of peptides and gradually increase your usage as your skin builds tolerance. This approach helps to minimize the risk of irritation while allowing your skin to fully benefit from the anti-aging properties of peptides.

In addition to topical skincare products, peptides are also being explored in other anti-aging treatments, such as injectable fillers and microneedling. Injectable fillers that contain peptides can provide more immediate results by delivering these powerful ingredients directly into the skin, where they can stimulate collagen production and enhance skin firmness. Microneedling, a procedure that creates tiny micro-injuries in the skin to stimulate collagen production, can be combined with peptide serums to further enhance the treatment's anti-aging effects.

As we continue to learn more about the science of aging and skin health, peptides will likely play an increasingly important role in anti-aging skincare. Their ability to target multiple aspects of skin aging—collagen production, moisture retention, and skin barrier function—makes them a versatile and valuable ingredient in the fight against aging. By incorporating peptides into your skincare routine, you can help to slow down the aging process, maintain a youthful appearance, and achieve healthier, more resilient skin.

2.3 Tyrosinase Inhibitors for Hyperpigmentation

Hyperpigmentation is a common skin concern characterized by dark spots or patches that appear due to an overproduction of melanin, the pigment responsible for skin color. These dark spots can result from various factors, including sun exposure, hormonal changes, aging, inflammation, or certain medications. One of the most effective ways to treat hyperpigmentation is through the use of tyrosinase inhibitors, which work by targeting the enzyme responsible for melanin production. Understanding how tyrosinase inhibitors function and how to incorporate them into a skincare routine can significantly improve skin tone and reduce the appearance of dark spots.

Tyrosinase is a copper-containing enzyme found in melanocytes, the cells that produce melanin. The role of tyrosinase in melanin production begins with its involvement in the conversion of tyrosine, an amino acid, into melanin. When tyrosinase activity increases, more melanin is produced, leading to hyperpigmentation. Tyrosinase inhibitors work by blocking the activity of this enzyme, thereby reducing melanin production and preventing new dark spots from forming.

Hydroquinone is one of the most widely recognized and effective tyrosinase inhibitors. It has been used for decades to lighten dark spots and even out skin tone. Hydroquinone works by directly inhibiting the activity of tyrosinase, reducing the formation of melanin and gradually lightening areas of hyperpigmentation. Due to its potency, hydroquinone is often recommended for stubborn cases of hyperpigmentation, such as melasma or post-inflammatory hyperpigmentation (PIH). However, hydroquinone can cause irritation and is not suitable for long-term use due to potential side effects, such as ochronosis, a rare condition that results in blue-black pigmentation. For this reason, it is typically used under the guidance of a dermatologist and is often cycled with other treatments to minimize side effects.

Kojic acid is another popular tyrosinase inhibitor derived from various fungi, including Aspergillus and Penicillium species. Kojic acid inhibits the action of tyrosinase by chelating the copper ions in the enzyme, which are essential for its activity. Kojic acid not only helps to lighten dark spots but also provides antioxidant benefits, protecting the skin from oxidative stress that can further exacerbate hyperpigmentation. Kojic acid is generally well-tolerated by most skin types, but some individuals may experience mild irritation or sensitivity, especially when used in higher concentrations. To minimize potential irritation, it is often combined with soothing ingredients like aloe vera or niacinamide.

Arbutin is a natural derivative of hydroquinone that is found in plants such as bearberry, cranberry, and blueberry. It is a milder alternative to hydroquinone and works similarly by inhibiting tyrosinase activity to prevent melanin production. Arbutin is particularly effective in treating sun-induced hyperpigmentation and melasma. Its gentle nature makes it suitable for all skin types, including sensitive skin, and it can be used for extended periods without the risks associated with hydroquinone. Alpha-arbutin, a more stable and potent form of arbutin, is often included in skincare products due to its higher efficacy in reducing dark spots and evening out skin tone.

Vitamin C is a potent antioxidant that also functions as a tyrosinase inhibitor. It interferes with melanin synthesis by reducing the activity of the enzyme and promoting a more even distribution of melanin in the skin. This dual action not only lightens existing dark spots but also protects the skin from further pigmentation caused by free radical damage. Vitamin C is effective in treating various types of hyperpigmentation, including age spots and sun damage, and is often used in combination with other tyrosinase inhibitors to enhance its brightening effects. It is important to note that vitamin C can be unstable and prone to oxidation, so it should be stored properly and used promptly to ensure maximum effectiveness.

Licorice root extract is a natural tyrosinase inhibitor that has gained popularity for its ability to brighten skin and reduce pigmentation. The active component in licorice root, glabridin, inhibits tyrosinase activity and has anti-inflammatory properties that help soothe irritated skin. This makes licorice root extract an excellent choice for individuals with sensitive skin who are looking to reduce hyperpigmentation without the risk of irritation. It is often found in brightening serums and creams designed to target dark spots and even out skin tone.

Niacinamide, also known as vitamin B3, is a versatile skincare ingredient that offers multiple benefits, including its role as a tyrosinase inhibitor. Niacinamide reduces the transfer of melanin to the surface of the skin, helping to prevent the appearance of new dark spots. Additionally, niacinamide has anti-inflammatory properties that can help reduce redness and irritation associated with hyperpigmentation. Its ability to improve the skin barrier function makes it suitable for use in various formulations, from serums to creams, and it is often combined with other tyrosinase inhibitors for a comprehensive approach to treating hyperpigmentation.

Azelaic acid is a naturally occurring acid found in grains like barley, wheat, and rye. It has mild exfoliating properties and works as a tyrosinase inhibitor by reducing the activity of melanocytes, the cells responsible for producing melanin. Azelaic acid is particularly effective in treating post-inflammatory hyperpigmentation (PIH), which is common among individuals with acne-prone skin. It helps to prevent the formation of new dark spots while also promoting a more even skin tone. Azelaic acid is gentle enough for sensitive skin and can be used in conjunction with other acne treatments to address both acne and PIH simultaneously.

Combining tyrosinase inhibitors can provide a synergistic effect, enhancing their overall efficacy in treating hyperpigmentation. For example, combining vitamin C with niacinamide or kojic acid can improve the brightening effect and reduce oxidative stress on the skin. Similarly, products containing a mix of arbutin, licorice root extract, and azelaic acid can target multiple pathways in melanin production, offering a more comprehensive solution for uneven skin tone and dark spots.

When using tyrosinase inhibitors, it is essential to incorporate them into a broader skincare routine that includes sun protection. Sun exposure can exacerbate hyperpigmentation, counteracting the effects of tyrosinase inhibitors. Therefore, using a broad-spectrum sunscreen with at least SPF 30 is crucial for protecting the skin from UV radiation and preventing new dark spots from forming. Additionally, incorporating hydrating and soothing ingredients, such as hyaluronic acid and ceramides, can help support the skin barrier and reduce any potential irritation caused by tyrosinase inhibitors.

It's important to be patient when using tyrosinase inhibitors, as visible results can take time to develop. The skin's natural turnover cycle is typically around 28 days, but it may take longer for dark spots to fade, especially if the pigmentation is deep or has been present for a long time. Consistent use of tyrosinase inhibitors, combined with a comprehensive skincare routine, is key to achieving the best results in treating hyperpigmentation.

Individuals with sensitive skin or those new to tyrosinase inhibitors should start with lower concentrations and gradually increase usage to assess their skin's tolerance. If any irritation or sensitivity occurs, it is advisable to reduce the frequency of use or consult a dermatologist for guidance on how to adjust the skincare regimen.

Overall, tyrosinase inhibitors are a valuable tool in the fight against hyperpigmentation and dark spots. By understanding their mechanisms of action and selecting the right products for your skin type and concerns, you can effectively reduce the appearance of hyperpigmentation and achieve a more even, radiant complexion.

2.4 Stem Cells in Skincare

Stem cells have emerged as a groundbreaking component in advanced skincare treatments, offering significant regenerative benefits that can enhance skin health and appearance. Their ability to self-renew and differentiate into various cell types makes them a valuable tool in promoting skin rejuvenation and addressing the signs of aging. In skincare, stem cells are primarily used for their potent regenerative properties, which help repair damaged skin, stimulate new cell growth, and improve the overall texture and tone of the skin.

Stem cells are unique because they have the potential to develop into different cell types and can also renew themselves by dividing. This characteristic is particularly important in skincare, where the goal is often to replace or repair damaged skin cells and to stimulate the production of new, healthy cells. In the context of skincare, stem cells do not replace human stem cells but rather support the skin's natural repair mechanisms. The most common types of stem cells used in skincare products are plant stem cells, animal stem cells, and human stem cell extracts.

Plant stem cells are the most frequently used in skincare due to their ethical appeal and effectiveness. These stem cells are derived from various parts of plants, including leaves, roots, and flowers, and are known for their antioxidant properties. Plant stem cells contain high levels of epigenetic factors and metabolites, which help protect the skin from environmental stressors, reduce inflammation, and promote cellular regeneration. For instance, apple stem cells, derived from a rare Swiss apple variety, are known for their ability to boost the longevity of skin cells and improve the appearance of fine lines and wrinkles. Similarly, grape stem cells are rich in polyphenols, which offer potent antioxidant protection against UV radiation and environmental damage.

Animal stem cells, particularly those derived from marine organisms like sea fennel, are also used in skincare for their regenerative properties. These stem cells are believed to promote cell turnover and enhance the skin's natural barrier function, making them beneficial for maintaining skin hydration and reducing the appearance of fine lines. While animal stem cells offer promising benefits, they are less commonly used due to ethical concerns and the increasing preference for plant-based ingredients in skincare.

Human stem cell extracts are derived from adult stem cells, typically obtained from fat or bone marrow tissue. These extracts contain growth factors and cytokines that are known to stimulate collagen production, promote wound healing, and improve skin elasticity. In skincare, human stem cell extracts are used to enhance the skin's ability to regenerate and repair itself, making them particularly effective in anti-aging treatments. These extracts are often found in high-end serums and creams designed to target deep wrinkles, sagging skin, and other advanced signs of aging. The use of human stem cell extracts in skincare is often limited to professional treatments offered in clinical settings, as they require stringent regulatory compliance and oversight.

The regenerative benefits of stem cells in skincare are primarily due to their ability to stimulate the production of collagen and elastin, the two proteins that provide structural support to the skin. Collagen is responsible for the skin's firmness and strength, while elastin allows the skin to return to its original shape after stretching or contracting. As we age, the natural production of these proteins declines, leading to the development of wrinkles, sagging skin, and loss of elasticity. Stem cells help counteract these effects by promoting the production of new collagen and elastin fibers, thereby improving the skin's overall texture and tone.

Stem cells also play a crucial role in protecting the skin from oxidative stress, which is a major contributor to the aging process. Oxidative stress occurs when there is an imbalance between free radicals and antioxidants in the body, leading to cellular damage. Stem cells, particularly those derived from plants, are rich in antioxidants that help neutralize free radicals and reduce oxidative damage to the skin. This protective effect is essential for maintaining a youthful appearance and preventing the formation of age spots, fine lines, and wrinkles.

In addition to their anti-aging benefits, stem cells are also effective in treating a variety of skin conditions, including acne, rosacea, and hyperpigmentation. For instance, stem cells can help reduce inflammation and promote healing in acne-prone skin, making them an excellent addition to treatments aimed at reducing breakouts and preventing scarring. Similarly, stem cells can help lighten dark spots and even out skin tone by promoting cellular turnover and reducing the appearance of hyperpigmentation.

One of the most significant advantages of stem cells in skincare is their ability to enhance the skin's natural barrier function. The skin barrier, also known as the stratum corneum, is the outermost layer of the skin that protects against environmental aggressors, retains moisture, and prevents the entry of harmful substances. A compromised skin barrier can lead to dryness, sensitivity, and an increased risk of infections. Stem cells help strengthen the skin barrier by promoting the production of lipids and proteins that are essential for maintaining its integrity. This not only helps to keep the skin hydrated and plump but also reduces the risk of irritation and inflammation.

To maximize the benefits of stem cells in skincare, it is important to use products that are formulated with high-quality, stable stem cell extracts. The effectiveness of stem cells in skincare largely depends on their stability and bioavailability, which can be influenced by the formulation and delivery system used. For example, encapsulation technology is often used to protect stem cell extracts from degradation and ensure their optimal delivery to the skin. Additionally, combining stem cells with other active ingredients, such as hyaluronic acid, peptides, and antioxidants, can further enhance their regenerative effects and provide a more comprehensive approach to skincare.

While stem cells offer numerous benefits for skin health and rejuvenation, it is important to note that their use in skincare is still a relatively new area of research. As such, consumers should approach stem cell-based products with a critical eye and seek out products that are backed by scientific evidence and clinical studies. Consulting with a dermatologist or skincare professional can also help determine whether stem cell-based treatments are appropriate for your skin type and concerns.

Incorporating stem cells into a skincare routine can provide significant anti-aging and regenerative benefits, particularly for individuals looking to address advanced signs of aging, improve skin texture, and promote a more youthful appearance. By understanding the role of stem cells in skincare and choosing products that are formulated with high-quality extracts, you can enhance your skin's natural ability to regenerate and repair itself, achieving healthier, more resilient skin.

2.5 Natural Ingredients and Eco-Sustainability

The demand for natural and eco-friendly skincare products has surged in recent years as consumers become more conscious of the ingredients they apply to their skin and the environmental impact of their choices. Natural ingredients, often derived from plants, minerals, and other naturally occurring substances, are prized for their gentle, bio-compatible properties that align with the skin's natural functions. Moreover, an emphasis on sustainability in skincare reflects a growing awareness of the need to protect the environment while nurturing personal health and well-being. Understanding the benefits of natural ingredients and their role in sustainable skincare can help consumers make more informed decisions that benefit both their skin and the planet.

Natural ingredients are derived from renewable resources, such as plants, fruits, seeds, and minerals. Unlike synthetic ingredients, which are often created through chemical processes, natural ingredients are harvested and processed with minimal intervention, retaining their inherent properties and benefits. These ingredients are often rich in vitamins, antioxidants, and essential fatty acids, which help nourish and protect the skin. For example, plant-based oils like jojoba, argan, and rosehip are known for their moisturizing and anti-inflammatory properties, making them ideal for soothing dry or irritated skin. Similarly, botanical extracts such as green tea, chamomile, and aloe vera provide antioxidant protection and help calm sensitive skin.

One of the primary advantages of natural ingredients is their bio-compatibility with the skin. Bio-compatibility refers to the ability of a substance to interact with the skin without causing irritation or adverse reactions. Because natural ingredients are often similar to the skin's own composition, they are more easily recognized and accepted by the skin. This reduces the likelihood of allergic reactions or sensitivities, making natural ingredients particularly beneficial for those with sensitive or reactive skin. Ingredients like calendula, shea butter, and oatmeal are renowned for their gentle, soothing properties and are frequently used in formulations designed for sensitive skin.

In addition to their compatibility with the skin, natural ingredients offer a holistic approach to skincare by addressing multiple concerns simultaneously. For instance, honey is a natural humectant that draws moisture into the skin, while also possessing antibacterial properties that can help treat acne. Similarly, turmeric, a spice commonly used in natural skincare, contains curcumin, which has anti-inflammatory and brightening effects, making it useful for treating hyperpigmentation and dullness. This multi-functional approach reduces the need for multiple products, simplifying skincare routines and minimizing the risk of product overload on the skin.

Eco-sustainability in skincare goes beyond the ingredients themselves and extends to the sourcing, production, and packaging of skincare products. Sustainable skincare practices prioritize the ethical sourcing of ingredients, ensuring that they are harvested in a way that does not deplete natural resources or harm local ecosystems. For example, ingredients like shea butter and argan oil are often sourced through fair-trade practices that support local communities and promote environmental conservation. By choosing products made with sustainably sourced ingredients, consumers can support efforts to protect biodiversity and promote sustainable farming practices.

The production process of natural skincare products also plays a critical role in sustainability. Many conventional skincare products are produced using processes that generate significant waste and pollution. In contrast, sustainable skincare brands focus on minimizing their environmental footprint by using energy-efficient production methods, reducing waste, and recycling materials whenever possible. Some brands even use upcycled ingredients—by-products of other industries that would otherwise go to waste, such as fruit seeds or coffee grounds—to create effective skincare products. This approach not only reduces waste but also adds value to ingredients that might otherwise be discarded.

Packaging is another important aspect of sustainable skincare. Traditional skincare products often come in single-use plastic containers that contribute to the growing problem of plastic pollution. Sustainable skincare brands, however, are increasingly adopting eco-friendly packaging solutions, such as recyclable glass, biodegradable materials, and refillable containers. These packaging options help reduce waste and encourage consumers to adopt more environmentally friendly habits. Some brands also use minimal packaging to reduce their environmental impact further, focusing on functionality and sustainability rather than elaborate designs.

The shift towards natural and sustainable skincare is also driven by a desire to avoid potentially harmful chemicals commonly found in conventional products. Ingredients like parabens, sulfates, phthalates, and synthetic fragrances are often criticized for their potential to cause skin irritation, disrupt hormones, or harm the environment. Natural skincare products, on the other hand, are formulated without these chemicals, offering a safer alternative for consumers looking to reduce their exposure to toxins. For example, natural preservatives like vitamin E and rosemary extract can be used to maintain product freshness without the need for synthetic additives.

However, it is important to note that not all natural ingredients are automatically safe or effective. Just because an ingredient is derived from a natural source does not mean it is free from the potential to cause irritation or allergic reactions. Essential oils, for example, are natural but can be highly concentrated and irritating if not used properly. Similarly, some plant extracts can cause photosensitivity, making the skin more susceptible to sun damage. Therefore, consumers should still exercise caution and conduct patch tests when trying new natural products, especially if they have sensitive or allergy-prone skin.

The integration of natural ingredients and eco-sustainability into skincare routines reflects a broader trend towards conscious consumerism. As consumers become more educated about the impact of their choices on their health and the environment, they are increasingly seeking products that align with their values. This shift is encouraging skincare brands to innovate and develop formulations that are not only effective but also ethical and sustainable. Brands that prioritize transparency about their sourcing, production methods, and ingredient lists are gaining trust and loyalty from consumers who are mindful of their ecological footprint.

Adopting a sustainable skincare routine involves not only selecting products made with natural and eco-friendly ingredients but also considering the overall impact of one's skincare habits. This might include using less water during cleansing, reducing the frequency of product application to avoid overuse, and choosing multi-functional products that reduce the need for multiple items. Additionally, consumers can look for certifications such as Fair Trade, USDA Organic, and Leaping Bunny to ensure that the products they purchase meet specific sustainability and ethical standards.

As the beauty industry continues to evolve, the focus on natural ingredients and eco-sustainability is likely to increase. Consumers are recognizing that skincare is not just about achieving beautiful skin but also about making responsible choices that support personal well-being and environmental health. By choosing natural, bio-compatible ingredients and supporting sustainable practices, individuals can contribute to a healthier planet while enhancing their skincare regimen.

CHAPTER 3: BUILDING YOUR SKINCARE ROUTINE

3.1 Personalizing Your Routine

Creating a personalized skincare routine is essential for achieving and maintaining healthy, radiant skin. A one-size-fits-all approach does not work in skincare because each individual's skin has unique characteristics, needs, and challenges. To design an effective skincare regimen, it is crucial to consider your skin type, specific concerns, and environmental factors that may affect your skin. A tailored routine helps address these unique needs, providing targeted care that enhances your skin's health and appearance.

The first step in personalizing your skincare routine is identifying your skin type. The four main skin types—normal, dry, oily, and combination—each have distinct characteristics and require different approaches. Normal skin is balanced and neither too oily nor too dry. A routine for normal skin focuses on maintaining this balance with gentle cleansing, regular moisturizing, and sun protection. Products with antioxidants and mild exfoliants can help keep the skin looking fresh and prevent early signs of aging.

Dry skin lacks sufficient moisture and oil, leading to a rough, flaky texture and a feeling of tightness. The primary goal for a dry skin routine is to replenish and retain moisture. This involves using a hydrating cleanser that does not strip the skin of its natural oils, followed by a rich moisturizer containing ingredients like hyaluronic acid, glycerin, and ceramides to lock in hydration. Incorporating a nourishing facial oil or balm can provide an additional moisture barrier, particularly in harsh weather conditions. Regular use of a hydrating mask can also help to boost the skin's moisture levels.

Oily skin is characterized by excess sebum production, which can lead to a shiny complexion, enlarged pores, and a propensity for acne. For oily skin, the routine should aim to control oil production without over-drying the skin, which can lead to increased oil production as a compensatory mechanism. A gentle foaming or gel cleanser that removes excess oil is ideal, followed by a lightweight, oil-free moisturizer to maintain hydration without clogging pores. Exfoliation with salicylic acid can help to keep pores clear and reduce breakouts. Clay masks are also beneficial for absorbing excess oil and refining the skin's texture.

Combination skin displays characteristics of both oily and dry skin, typically with an oily T-zone (forehead, nose, and chin) and drier or normal skin on the cheeks. The key to managing combination skin is to balance the varying needs of different areas of the face. A gentle, pH-balanced cleanser works well to clean the entire face without causing dryness or excess oil production. Using a lightweight, hydrating moisturizer for the entire face and applying an oil-controlling product on the T-zone can help maintain balance. Multi-masking—using different masks on different parts of the face—is also effective for treating the specific needs of combination skin.

Once your skin type is determined, the next step is to identify specific skin concerns. Common concerns include acne, hyperpigmentation, sensitivity, and aging. Each of these issues requires targeted ingredients and treatments to achieve the best results. For acne-prone skin, products containing salicylic acid, benzoyl peroxide, or retinoids can help reduce breakouts by keeping pores clear and promoting cell turnover. For hyperpigmentation, ingredients such as vitamin C, niacinamide, and tyrosinase inhibitors like kojic acid or arbutin are effective in lightening dark spots and evening out skin tone.

Sensitive skin needs a routine that focuses on soothing and protecting the skin barrier. Avoiding harsh exfoliants, fragrances, and alcohol is crucial for minimizing irritation. Gentle cleansers, hydrating serums, and moisturizers with ingredients like aloe vera, chamomile, and ceramides can help calm the skin and reduce redness. For anti-aging concerns, ingredients like retinoids, peptides, and antioxidants are effective in promoting collagen production, reducing fine lines, and improving skin elasticity.

Environmental factors also play a significant role in shaping a personalized skincare routine. Climate, pollution levels, and even stress can affect how your skin behaves and responds to different products. In hot and humid climates, the skin tends to produce more oil, which can lead to clogged pores and breakouts. In these conditions, a lighter routine with oil-free products and regular use of exfoliants can help manage excess oil. In contrast, colder climates with low humidity can exacerbate dryness and flakiness, requiring a richer, more emollient routine to protect and hydrate the skin.

Pollution can lead to oxidative stress, which accelerates skin aging and triggers inflammation. Incorporating antioxidants like vitamin C, E, and green tea into your routine can help neutralize free radicals caused by pollution. Additionally, thorough cleansing is essential to remove pollutants that can clog pores and damage the skin barrier. If you live in an area with high pollution, consider double cleansing with a gentle oil-based cleanser followed by a foaming or cream cleanser to ensure all impurities are removed.

Stress can also impact the skin, leading to issues like breakouts, redness, and increased sensitivity. A personalized skincare routine should include products that help strengthen the skin barrier and reduce inflammation, such as niacinamide, peptides, and soothing botanicals. Incorporating self-care practices, such as facial massage or a calming mask, can also help alleviate stress and improve overall skin health.

To create a truly personalized skincare routine, it is essential to consider not only your skin type and concerns but also your lifestyle and preferences. A routine should be sustainable and enjoyable, tailored to fit seamlessly into your daily life. If you have limited time, focusing on multi-functional products that address multiple concerns can simplify your routine without compromising efficacy. For those who enjoy a more elaborate routine, layering serums and treatments with different active ingredients can provide a more targeted approach.

Tracking your skin's progress over time is also important in a personalized skincare routine. Skin can change due to factors like age, hormonal shifts, and seasonal variations, so it is crucial to remain flexible and adjust your routine as needed. Keeping a skincare journal or taking regular photos can help you monitor changes in your skin's condition and identify patterns or triggers that affect your skin health.

A personalized skincare routine is a dynamic process that evolves with your skin's needs. By understanding your skin type, identifying specific concerns, and considering environmental and lifestyle factors, you can create a routine that enhances your skin's natural beauty and supports its health. With consistent care and attention, a personalized routine can help you achieve and maintain radiant, healthy skin at any age.

3.2 Effective Cleansing

Cleansing is the cornerstone of any skincare routine, as it removes dirt, oil, makeup, and environmental pollutants that accumulate on the skin throughout the day. Effective cleansing not only keeps the skin clean but also prepares it for subsequent skincare steps, ensuring that active ingredients in serums and moisturizers can penetrate more deeply and work more effectively. However, cleansing is not a one-size-fits-all process. The choice of cleanser and method must be tailored to your skin type and specific needs to maintain a healthy balance and prevent irritation or dryness.

Cleansers come in various formulations, each designed to address different skin types and concerns. The most common types include gel cleansers, cream cleansers, foam cleansers, oil cleansers, and micellar water. Each type has distinct properties that make it suitable for specific skin conditions, and understanding these differences is crucial for choosing the right product for your skin.

Gel Cleansers are typically clear, water-based formulas designed for deep cleansing. They are particularly effective for oily and acne-prone skin types because they can penetrate deeply into pores to remove excess oil, bacteria, and impurities without leaving a heavy residue. Gel cleansers often contain exfoliating acids like salicylic acid or glycolic acid, which help to unclog pores and prevent breakouts. These cleansers are excellent for removing makeup and environmental pollutants that can lead to skin congestion. However, they may not be the best choice for dry or sensitive skin, as they can sometimes strip the skin of its natural oils, leading to dryness or irritation.

Cream Cleansers have a thicker, lotion-like texture that provides a more moisturizing cleanse. These cleansers are ideal for dry, mature, or sensitive skin types because they contain emollients that help to retain moisture while cleansing. Cream cleansers gently remove dirt and makeup without disrupting the skin's natural barrier, making them less likely to cause irritation. They often contain soothing ingredients like chamomile, aloe vera, or glycerin, which help to calm the skin and reduce redness. For those with dry or sensitive skin, cream cleansers can be an excellent option, particularly in colder months when the skin is more prone to dryness.

Foam Cleansers are lightweight formulas that create a foamy lather when mixed with water. They are often marketed for normal to combination skin types, as they effectively remove dirt, oil, and makeup without being too harsh. Foam cleansers can be a good choice for those who enjoy the sensation of a deep clean but want to avoid the drying effects of some gel cleansers. However, some foam cleansers can contain surfactants, such as sodium lauryl sulfate, which can strip the skin of its natural oils. It's important to choose a sulfate-free foam cleanser if you have sensitive or dry skin to avoid irritation and dryness.

Oil Cleansers use the principle of "like dissolves like," meaning that they use oils to break down and dissolve other oils on the skin. Oil cleansers are highly effective at removing waterproof makeup, sunscreen, and excess sebum without stripping the skin. They are particularly beneficial for dry or sensitive skin types, as they help maintain the skin's natural moisture barrier while providing a thorough cleanse. For those with oily or acne-prone skin, using an oil cleanser may seem counterintuitive, but when formulated with non-comedogenic oils like jojoba or grapeseed oil, they can effectively cleanse the skin without clogging pores. Oil cleansers are often used as the first step in a double-cleansing routine, followed by a water-based cleanser to remove any remaining residue.

Micellar Water is a no-rinse cleansing solution that uses micelles—tiny oil molecules suspended in soft water—to capture and lift away dirt, oil, and makeup. Micellar water is gentle and can be used on all skin types, including sensitive skin. It is particularly convenient for those who need a quick cleanse without access to water or for those with very sensitive skin that reacts to traditional cleansers. Micellar water can be an excellent option for a morning cleanse or as a pre-cleanse before using a more targeted cleanser at night. However, it may not be sufficient on its own for removing heavy makeup or sunscreen. When choosing a cleanser, it's important to consider not only your skin type but also the specific needs and conditions your skin is currently facing. For example, if your skin is oily but dehydrated, you might benefit from a gentle gel cleanser that cleanses without stripping essential moisture. If your skin is dry and prone to irritation, a cream or oil cleanser that provides hydration and soothing benefits would be more appropriate.

The method of cleansing is equally important in achieving effective results. **Double cleansing** is a popular technique that involves using two types of cleansers: an oil-based cleanser to remove makeup, sunscreen, and excess oil, followed by a water-based cleanser to cleanse deeper impurities and residue. This method is particularly beneficial for those who wear heavy makeup or live in areas with high pollution levels. Double cleansing ensures that all traces of dirt and impurities are thoroughly removed, allowing for better absorption of skincare products that follow.

Massage techniques during cleansing can also enhance the effectiveness of the process. Massaging the cleanser into the skin using gentle, circular motions helps to increase blood circulation and stimulate lymphatic drainage, which can reduce puffiness and promote a healthy glow. Additionally, massaging the skin helps to dislodge dirt and debris from the pores more effectively than a quick wash. Spending a few extra seconds on each area of the face can make a noticeable difference in the cleanliness and health of the skin.

Temperature plays a crucial role in the cleansing process. Using water that is too hot can strip the skin of its natural oils, leading to dryness and irritation, while water that is too cold may not effectively dissolve oils and dirt. Lukewarm water is the ideal temperature for cleansing, as it helps to open the pores slightly without causing damage or dehydration. After cleansing, a splash of cool water can help to close the pores and give the skin a refreshed feeling.

It's also essential to consider the **frequency of cleansing**. While cleansing twice a day—once in the morning and once at night—is a common recommendation, the needs may vary depending on your skin type and lifestyle. For example, individuals with very dry or sensitive skin may find that cleansing only once a day, preferably at night, is sufficient to avoid over-stripping the skin. On the other hand, those with oily or acne-prone skin may benefit from a more consistent cleansing routine to keep excess oil and impurities under control.

Finally, it's crucial to **evaluate the ingredients** in your chosen cleanser. Look for cleansers that are free from harsh sulfates, parabens, and synthetic fragrances, which can irritate the skin and compromise the skin barrier. Instead, opt for products that include nourishing and hydrating ingredients, such as hyaluronic acid, ceramides, and botanical extracts, which can help maintain the skin's natural balance while providing effective cleansing.

Effective cleansing is the foundation of a good skincare routine. By choosing the right cleanser for your skin type and needs, using the correct techniques, and considering factors such as water temperature and frequency, you can achieve a thorough, gentle cleanse that prepares your skin for the rest of your skincare regimen. Whether you opt for a gel, cream, foam, oil, or micellar water cleanser, the key is to ensure that your cleansing routine supports your skin's overall health and enhances the efficacy of the products that follow.

3.3 Exfoliation: Chemical vs. Physical

Exfoliation is a key step in any effective skincare routine, as it removes dead skin cells that can accumulate on the surface, leading to a dull complexion, clogged pores, and uneven texture. Regular exfoliation helps to reveal fresher, healthier skin beneath, promotes cell turnover, and enhances the absorption of skincare products. There are two main types of exfoliation: chemical and physical. Each method offers unique benefits and should be chosen based on skin type, concerns, and personal preference.

Chemical exfoliation involves the use of acids or enzymes to dissolve the bonds that hold dead skin cells together, allowing them to be easily sloughed away. This type of exfoliation is generally more uniform and controlled than physical exfoliation, making it suitable for a wide range of skin types, including sensitive and acne-prone skin. Chemical exfoliants are typically divided into two categories: alpha hydroxy acids (AHAs) and beta hydroxy acids (BHAs).

Alpha hydroxy acids (AHAs) are water-soluble acids derived from fruits and milk. Common AHAs include glycolic acid, lactic acid, mandelic acid, and citric acid. AHAs work on the surface of the skin to exfoliate the uppermost layers, making them particularly effective for addressing issues like dullness, uneven skin tone, and fine lines. Glycolic acid, derived from sugar cane, is the smallest molecule among the AHAs, allowing it to penetrate the skin effectively and provide noticeable results. However, its potency can also increase the risk of irritation, especially for those with sensitive skin. Lactic acid, derived from milk, is a milder AHA that provides similar benefits with less risk of irritation, making it suitable for more sensitive skin types.

Beta hydroxy acids (BHAs) are oil-soluble acids, with salicylic acid being the most common BHA used in skincare. BHAs are able to penetrate deeper into the pores, making them particularly effective for oily and acne-prone skin. Salicylic acid exfoliates the surface of the skin while also dissolving sebum within the pores, helping to prevent and treat blackheads, whiteheads, and acne. BHAs also have anti-inflammatory and antibacterial properties, which further help in reducing acne-related redness and swelling.

Enzyme exfoliants are another form of chemical exfoliation derived from natural sources such as papaya (papain) and pineapple (bromelain). These enzymes work by breaking down the keratin protein in the dead skin cells, leading to gentle exfoliation. Enzyme exfoliants are typically less irritating than AHAs and BHAs, making them an excellent choice for sensitive skin types or those new to exfoliation.

Physical exfoliation involves manually scrubbing away dead skin cells using a product containing small, gritty particles, such as sugar, salt, coffee grounds, or jojoba beads, or using tools like brushes, sponges, or microfiber cloths. Physical exfoliants provide immediate results, as the act of scrubbing helps to physically remove dead skin cells from the surface. They can also improve circulation and promote lymphatic drainage, leading to a temporary brightening and tightening effect on the skin.

While physical exfoliation can be effective, it requires careful use to avoid over-exfoliation or irritation. Over-scrubbing or using abrasive materials can cause microtears in the skin, leading to increased sensitivity, redness, and even potential long-term damage. For this reason, it is crucial to choose a gentle physical exfoliant with fine, rounded particles that will not scratch or damage the skin. Those with normal to oily skin may benefit from physical exfoliation, while individuals with sensitive, dry, or acne-prone skin should use caution or opt for gentler alternatives.

When deciding between chemical and physical exfoliation, it is important to consider your skin type and specific concerns. Chemical exfoliation tends to be more controlled and can provide a more uniform exfoliation without the risk of abrasion, making it suitable for most skin types, including sensitive and acne-prone skin. AHAs are ideal for those dealing with dry skin, hyperpigmentation, or fine lines, while BHAs are better suited for oily, acne-prone skin. Enzyme exfoliants offer a gentle option for sensitive skin or those new to exfoliation.

For those who prefer immediate results or have normal to oily skin, physical exfoliation can be an effective option. However, it should be done with caution to avoid over-exfoliating or irritating the skin. Using a soft washcloth, a konjac sponge, or a gentle scrub with rounded particles can help to provide effective physical exfoliation without damaging the skin barrier.

Guidelines for Safe and Effective Exfoliation

To exfoliate safely and effectively, it is important to follow a few key guidelines:

1. **Choose the Right Exfoliant for Your Skin Type:** Select an exfoliant that is suitable for your skin type and concerns. For example, if you have sensitive skin, opt for

a gentle AHA like lactic acid or an enzyme exfoliant. If you have oily, acne-prone skin, consider using a BHA like salicylic acid.

2. **Start Slowly and Gradually Increase Frequency:** When introducing a new exfoliant into your routine, start slowly to assess your skin's tolerance. Begin with once or twice a week and gradually increase the frequency as your skin builds tolerance. Over-exfoliation can lead to irritation, redness, and a compromised skin barrier.

3. **Pay Attention to Your Skin's Response:** Monitor your skin's response to the exfoliant and adjust the frequency or type of exfoliation if you notice any signs of irritation, redness, or increased sensitivity. It is important to listen to your skin and give it time to adjust to new products.

4. **Avoid Overlapping Exfoliants:** Avoid using multiple exfoliating products in the same routine or using them too frequently, as this can lead to over-exfoliation and damage to the skin barrier. If you use an AHA or BHA serum, skip the physical scrub to prevent irritation.

5. **Use Sun Protection:** Exfoliation can make the skin more sensitive to the sun, so it is crucial to apply broad-spectrum sunscreen with at least SPF 30 during the day. Sun protection helps to prevent sunburn, hyperpigmentation, and other sun-related damage, especially after exfoliation.

6. **Incorporate Hydration and Barrier-Repair Ingredients:** After exfoliating, follow up with hydrating and soothing products to restore moisture and support the skin barrier. Ingredients like hyaluronic acid, ceramides, and glycerin can help maintain the skin's hydration and repair any potential damage caused by exfoliation.

7. **Be Mindful of Other Skincare Products:** Certain skincare ingredients, such as retinoids, can increase skin sensitivity and should not be combined with strong exfoliants. When using multiple active ingredients, space them out in your routine to minimize irritation.

Exfoliation is a powerful tool in maintaining healthy, radiant skin, but it must be approached with care. By understanding the differences between chemical and physical exfoliation and following safe exfoliation practices, you can achieve a smoother, brighter complexion without compromising your skin's health. Whether you choose a chemical exfoliant like an AHA or BHA, or a gentle physical exfoliant, the key is to tailor your approach to your skin's needs and avoid over-exfoliation to maintain a balanced, glowing complexion.

3.4 Hydration: Myths and Realities

Hydration is a fundamental component of any effective skincare routine, but it is often misunderstood. Proper hydration is not just about drinking water; it involves using the right skincare products to maintain and enhance the skin's natural moisture levels. Hydrated skin is more resilient, appears plumper, and has a healthy glow. However, with so many myths surrounding hydration and the vast array of moisturizers available, it is important to understand the science behind skin hydration, the types of moisturizers, and how to choose the right one for your skin's specific needs.

One common myth is that oily skin does not need hydration. Many people with oily skin believe that using a moisturizer will make their skin more greasy and prone to breakouts. However, oily skin can still be dehydrated, lacking water rather than oil. Dehydrated skin can produce even more oil in an attempt to compensate for the lack of moisture, leading to an overproduction of sebum and clogged pores. This is why even oily skin types need a good moisturizer that provides hydration without adding excess oil. Lightweight, oil-free moisturizers with ingredients like hyaluronic acid and glycerin are ideal for hydrating oily skin without clogging pores or making the skin feel heavy.

Another misconception is that drinking more water will instantly hydrate the skin. While staying hydrated is important for overall health and can have some impact on the skin, the direct effects of drinking water on skin hydration are minimal. The skin is the last organ to receive water from the body, so topical hydration is crucial for maintaining healthy skin. Topical hydrators, such as moisturizers, serums, and facial mists, provide immediate moisture to the skin's outer layers, helping to maintain a balanced moisture level and prevent dryness and irritation.

The skin's natural barrier, also known as the lipid barrier, plays a vital role in maintaining hydration. This barrier consists of lipids (fats) that help retain moisture and protect the skin from environmental aggressors. When this barrier is compromised, the skin loses moisture more rapidly, leading to dryness, irritation, and increased sensitivity. Effective hydration involves not only adding moisture to the skin but also supporting the lipid barrier to prevent moisture loss. Moisturizers containing ceramides, fatty acids, and cholesterol are particularly effective in reinforcing the skin barrier and locking in hydration.

There are several types of moisturizers, each formulated with different ingredients to target specific skin needs. **Humectants** are ingredients that attract water from the environment and draw it into the skin, helping to increase hydration levels. Common humectants include hyaluronic acid, glycerin, urea, and aloe vera. These ingredients are especially beneficial for dehydrated skin, as they provide lightweight hydration without a greasy feel. Hyaluronic acid, in particular, is known for its ability to hold up to 1,000 times its weight in water, making it a powerful hydrating agent that can be used by all skin types.

Emollients are moisturizing ingredients that soften and smooth the skin by filling in the gaps between skin cells, providing a temporary barrier to lock in moisture. Emollients are ideal for dry or mature skin types that need additional softness and suppleness. Ingredients like shea butter, squalane, and plant oils (such as jojoba, argan, and coconut oil) are commonly used as emollients in moisturizers. These ingredients help to improve the skin's texture and provide a barrier that prevents moisture loss while delivering essential fatty acids that nourish the skin.

Occlusives are thicker moisturizing agents that create a physical barrier on the surface of the skin to prevent water loss. They are particularly beneficial for very dry or compromised skin, as they provide an intense level of hydration and protection. Common occlusives include petrolatum, beeswax, lanolin, and silicones. These ingredients are especially effective in protecting the skin from harsh environmental conditions, such as cold weather or wind, which can exacerbate dryness. However, occlusives can feel heavy on the skin, so they are often used in conjunction with lighter moisturizers or applied at night to provide overnight hydration.

The choice of moisturizer should be guided by the skin's specific needs and the environment in which you live. For example, in a dry climate, the skin may require a more hydrating and protective moisturizer to combat the effects of low humidity and environmental stressors. In contrast, in a more humid climate, a lightweight, non-comedogenic moisturizer may be sufficient to maintain hydration without feeling greasy or clogging pores.

Sensitive skin requires a more cautious approach to hydration, as it is prone to reactions from fragrances, dyes, and certain preservatives found in many moisturizers. For sensitive skin, choosing a moisturizer with minimal ingredients and avoiding potential irritants is essential. Look for products labeled as "hypoallergenic" and those containing soothing ingredients like aloe vera, chamomile, and allantoin. These ingredients help to calm and protect sensitive skin while providing adequate hydration without causing irritation.

Mature skin, which often experiences a decrease in natural oil production and a thinning of the lipid barrier, benefits from richer, more nourishing moisturizers that provide both hydration and barrier support. Ingredients like peptides, retinoids, and antioxidants can be included in a mature skin moisturizer to provide anti-aging benefits while maintaining hydration. Products that combine humectants, emollients, and occlusives offer a comprehensive approach to hydration, helping to plump the skin, reduce the appearance of fine lines, and protect against environmental damage.

Dehydrated skin, which can occur in any skin type, needs a specific approach that focuses on increasing water content. A combination of a hydrating serum with hyaluronic acid followed by a lightweight moisturizer can help address dehydration without making the skin feel oily or heavy. Adding a facial mist throughout the day can also provide an instant boost of hydration and refresh the skin, especially in dry or air-conditioned environments.

When incorporating hydration into your skincare routine, it's important to apply products in the correct order to maximize their effectiveness. Start with a hydrating serum or essence, which is lighter and can penetrate deeper into the skin. Follow with a moisturizer that provides the right balance of hydration and barrier protection for your skin type. For those with very dry or compromised skin, adding an occlusive layer at night can help lock in moisture and repair the skin barrier while you sleep.

Hydration is essential for all skin types and is the foundation of healthy, balanced skin. By understanding the different types of moisturizers and how to choose the right one based on your skin's specific needs, you can create a hydration strategy that enhances your skin's natural beauty and resilience. With the right approach to hydration, you can achieve a complexion that looks and feels smooth, supple, and radiant.

3.5 Sunscreen: The Essential Element

Sunscreen is widely recognized as one of the most important components of any skincare routine, and for good reason. It plays a critical role in protecting the skin from the harmful effects of ultraviolet (UV) radiation, which can cause premature aging, sunburn, and increase the risk of skin cancer. Incorporating sunscreen into your daily routine is essential, regardless of skin type, age, or geographical location. To effectively protect your skin, it is important to understand the different types of sunscreens available, how they work, and the best practices for integrating them into your skincare regimen.

There are two main types of sunscreens: **chemical (organic) filters** and **physical (inorganic) filters**. Each type offers unique benefits and is formulated with different ingredients to protect the skin from UV radiation.

Chemical sunscreens contain organic compounds such as oxybenzone, avobenzone, octisalate, octocrylene, homosalate, and octinoxate. These compounds work by absorbing UV radiation and converting it into heat, which is then released from the skin. Chemical sunscreens typically provide broad-spectrum protection, meaning they guard against both UVA and UVB rays. UVA rays penetrate deep into the skin and are primarily responsible for premature aging and the development of fine lines and wrinkles, while UVB rays affect the outer layer of the skin, causing sunburn and contributing to skin cancer risk.

One of the advantages of chemical sunscreens is their lightweight texture, which absorbs quickly into the skin without leaving a white cast or greasy residue. This makes them an excellent choice for daily use under makeup or for those with darker skin tones, who may find physical sunscreens more challenging to blend. However, some chemical filters can cause irritation or allergic reactions, particularly for those with sensitive skin. Additionally, certain chemical sunscreens may degrade when exposed to sunlight, reducing their effectiveness over time. To mitigate this, many formulations include stabilizing ingredients or recommend reapplication every two hours, especially during prolonged sun exposure.

Physical sunscreens, also known as mineral sunscreens, use active ingredients such as zinc oxide and titanium dioxide to provide a physical barrier on the skin's surface. These ingredients reflect and scatter UV radiation, preventing it from penetrating the skin. Physical sunscreens are often recommended for individuals with sensitive skin, as they are less likely to cause irritation or allergic reactions. They provide broad-spectrum protection and are effective immediately upon application, making them a reliable option for those seeking immediate protection.

One of the primary benefits of physical sunscreens is their stability; they do not degrade when exposed to sunlight, maintaining their effectiveness for longer periods. However, physical sunscreens tend to have a thicker consistency and may leave a white cast on the skin, particularly on darker skin tones. Advances in formulation technology have led to the development of micronized and tinted versions, which help minimize this effect and improve aesthetic appeal.

When choosing a sunscreen, it is important to select one that offers broad-spectrum protection, with a sun protection factor (SPF) of at least 30. Broad-spectrum sunscreens protect against both UVA and UVB rays, while SPF indicates the level of protection against UVB rays. An SPF of 30 blocks approximately 97% of UVB rays, while higher SPF values provide slightly more protection. However, no sunscreen can block 100% of UV rays, making regular reapplication and other sun protection measures essential.

Incorporating sunscreen into your daily routine involves more than just applying it before heading outdoors. Sunscreen should be the final step in your morning skincare routine, applied after moisturizer but before makeup. To ensure adequate protection, apply a generous amount—about a quarter teaspoon for the face and neck and one ounce (a shot glass) for the entire body. It's important to apply sunscreen to all exposed areas, including the ears, neck, décolletage, and hands, as these areas are often overlooked but highly susceptible to sun damage.

Reapplication is key to maintaining effective sun protection throughout the day. Sunscreen should be reapplied every two hours when outdoors, or immediately after swimming, sweating, or towel drying. For those who wear makeup, reapplying sunscreen can be challenging. In these cases, powder or spray sunscreens can be a convenient option, providing a layer of protection without disrupting makeup. It is also advisable to carry a travel-sized sunscreen for touch-ups, especially during outdoor activities or extended exposure to sunlight.

While sunscreen is the most effective way to protect the skin from UV radiation, it should be part of a comprehensive sun protection strategy. This includes wearing protective clothing, such as wide-brimmed hats and UV-blocking sunglasses, seeking shade during peak sun hours (10 a.m. to 4 p.m.), and avoiding tanning beds, which emit harmful UV radiation. Additionally, antioxidants like vitamin C, vitamin E, and niacinamide can be incorporated into your skincare routine to provide additional protection against free radical damage caused by UV exposure.

There are several misconceptions about sunscreen that need to be addressed to ensure proper usage. One common myth is that sunscreen is only necessary on sunny days or during summer. UV radiation can penetrate clouds, and up to 80% of UV rays can pass through on cloudy days. Moreover, UV exposure can occur throughout the year, making daily sunscreen application essential, regardless of the weather or season. Another misconception is that those with darker skin tones do not need sunscreen. While melanin provides some natural protection against UV radiation, it does not eliminate the risk of sun damage or skin cancer. Everyone, regardless of skin tone, should use sunscreen to protect against harmful UV effects.

Some people are concerned about the potential health risks associated with certain sunscreen ingredients. While some studies have raised questions about the absorption of certain chemical filters into the bloodstream, the benefits of using sunscreen to prevent skin cancer and premature aging far outweigh these concerns. For those who prefer to avoid chemical filters, mineral sunscreens offer a safe and effective alternative without the associated risks.

Environmental impact is another consideration when choosing a sunscreen. Some chemical sunscreen ingredients, such as oxybenzone and octinoxate, have been linked to coral bleaching and harm to marine life. To reduce environmental impact, consider using reef-safe sunscreens, which do not contain harmful chemicals and are designed to be safe for both the skin and the ocean. Look for sunscreens labeled as "reef-safe" or "reef-friendly" and avoid products with harmful ingredients that can affect coral reefs and aquatic ecosystems.

Ultimately, the best sunscreen is the one you will use consistently. It should be suitable for your skin type, comfortable to wear, and easy to apply. Whether you choose a chemical or physical sunscreen, the key is to make it a non-negotiable part of your daily routine, just like brushing your teeth or washing your face. With regular use, sunscreen helps prevent the immediate and long-term effects of sun exposure, supporting healthier, more youthful-looking skin. By understanding the importance of sunscreen and integrating it effectively into your daily regimen, you can significantly reduce the risk of sun damage and enjoy radiant, protected skin all year round.

CHAPTER 4: ADVANCED TREATMENTS FOR SPECIFIC ISSUES

4.1 Acne: Understanding and Treating

Acne is one of the most common skin conditions, affecting millions of people worldwide, regardless of age, gender, or ethnicity. It occurs when hair follicles become clogged with oil, dead skin cells, and bacteria, leading to the formation of pimples, blackheads, whiteheads, cysts, or nodules. While acne is most prevalent during adolescence due to hormonal changes, it can persist into adulthood or develop for the first time in later years. Understanding the underlying causes of acne and the most effective treatment options is essential for managing breakouts and achieving clearer, healthier skin.

The primary cause of acne is the overproduction of sebum, an oily substance produced by the sebaceous glands. Sebum helps to protect and lubricate the skin, but when produced in excess, it can mix with dead skin cells and form a plug within the hair follicle, leading to clogged pores. Hormonal fluctuations, particularly an increase in androgens, can trigger this overproduction of sebum. This is why acne is so common during puberty, menstruation, pregnancy, and in conditions like polycystic ovary syndrome (PCOS). Hormones stimulate the sebaceous glands to produce more oil, creating an environment where acne-causing bacteria, such as *Propionibacterium acnes* (P. acnes), can thrive.

Another contributing factor to acne is the accumulation of dead skin cells. Normally, skin cells shed regularly, but when this process is disrupted, dead cells can accumulate on the skin's surface and within the pores, contributing to clogged follicles. This is particularly common in individuals with oily skin, as excess oil can cause skin cells to stick together and prevent proper shedding.

Inflammation plays a critical role in the development and severity of acne. When a pore becomes clogged and bacteria begin to proliferate, the body's immune response triggers inflammation in the surrounding tissue. This inflammation manifests as redness, swelling, and pus-filled lesions, commonly referred to as pimples or pustules. In more severe cases, the inflammation can penetrate deeper into the skin, leading to the formation of cysts or nodules, which are painful, larger lesions that can result in scarring.

To effectively manage and treat acne, it is essential to adopt a multi-faceted approach that targets each of these contributing factors. One of the most effective first-line treatments for acne is the use of topical retinoids, such as tretinoin, adapalene, and tazarotene. Retinoids are derivatives of vitamin A that work by increasing cell turnover, preventing the formation of clogged pores, and reducing inflammation. By promoting the shedding of dead skin cells and preventing their accumulation, retinoids help to keep pores clear and reduce the likelihood of breakouts. They also have anti-inflammatory properties that can help to calm existing lesions and reduce redness.

Topical retinoids are available in various strengths and formulations, making them suitable for different skin types and levels of acne severity. For those new to retinoids, it is advisable to start with a lower concentration and gradually increase the strength to allow the skin to build tolerance and minimize irritation. Applying retinoids at night, as part of an evening skincare routine, is recommended since they can make the skin more sensitive to sunlight.

Another cornerstone in acne treatment is the use of **benzoyl peroxide**, a powerful antibacterial agent that helps reduce the presence of *P. acnes* on the skin. Benzoyl peroxide works by introducing oxygen into the pores, creating an inhospitable environment for the anaerobic bacteria that thrive in oxygen-deprived conditions. This action helps to reduce inflammation and clear up existing acne lesions. Benzoyl peroxide is available in various concentrations, typically ranging from 2.5% to 10%. It can be used alone or in combination with other treatments, such as topical retinoids or antibiotics, for a more comprehensive approach.

While effective, benzoyl peroxide can be drying and irritating, especially for those with sensitive skin. To minimize potential side effects, it is important to start with a lower concentration and gradually increase usage as the skin builds tolerance. Additionally, moisturizing regularly and using a gentle cleanser can help to mitigate dryness and irritation associated with benzoyl peroxide use.

Salicylic acid is another popular treatment for acne, particularly for individuals with oily or combination skin. Salicylic acid is a beta hydroxy acid (BHA) that penetrates the pores and exfoliates from within, helping to remove dead skin cells and excess sebum that can lead to clogged pores. Its anti-inflammatory properties also make it effective in reducing redness and swelling associated with acne lesions. Salicylic acid is commonly found in cleansers, toners, and spot treatments, allowing for easy incorporation into a daily skincare routine.

For individuals with more severe or persistent acne, oral medications may be necessary to achieve optimal results. **Oral antibiotics**, such as doxycycline, minocycline, and tetracycline, are often prescribed to reduce the bacterial load on the skin and decrease inflammation. These antibiotics help control the growth of *P. acnes* and reduce the inflammatory response that contributes to acne severity. However, long-term use of antibiotics is not recommended due to the risk of antibiotic resistance and potential side effects. Oral antibiotics are typically used for a limited period, in conjunction with topical treatments, to achieve initial control of acne before transitioning to maintenance therapy.

Hormonal treatments can be particularly effective for women experiencing acne due to hormonal fluctuations. Birth control pills containing estrogen and progestin help regulate hormones and reduce the androgen levels that stimulate excess sebum production. Spironolactone, a medication that blocks androgen receptors, is another hormonal treatment that can be effective in reducing oil production and acne breakouts in women. These treatments require a prescription and should be discussed with a healthcare provider to determine their suitability and potential risks.

For cases of severe, cystic acne that do not respond to other treatments, **oral isotretinoin** (commonly known by the brand name Accutane) may be considered. Isotretinoin is a powerful retinoid that works by reducing the size and activity of the sebaceous glands, decreasing oil production, and promoting skin cell turnover. While highly effective in clearing severe acne, isotretinoin has a range of potential side effects, including dryness, increased sensitivity to sunlight, and, in rare cases, more serious health risks. Its use requires close monitoring by a healthcare professional, and patients must adhere to strict guidelines, including regular blood tests and pregnancy prevention measures.

In addition to medical treatments, certain lifestyle changes can also play a crucial role in managing acne. Maintaining a consistent skincare routine that includes gentle cleansing, exfoliation, and moisturizing can help keep the skin balanced and reduce the risk of breakouts. Avoiding harsh or abrasive skincare products that can irritate the skin and exacerbate acne is essential. Non-comedogenic products, which do not clog pores, are recommended for individuals prone to acne.

Diet and lifestyle can also influence acne. Some studies suggest that a diet high in refined sugars and dairy products may exacerbate acne in some individuals. Incorporating a balanced diet rich in fruits, vegetables, lean proteins, and whole grains can support overall skin health. Additionally, managing stress through relaxation techniques, such as meditation or exercise, can help reduce the hormonal fluctuations that may trigger or worsen acne.

Addressing acne scars is another important aspect of acne management, especially for those with a history of severe or cystic acne. Acne scars can take several forms, including atrophic scars (such as icepick, boxcar, and rolling scars), hypertrophic scars, and post-inflammatory hyperpigmentation (PIH). Treatment options for acne scars vary depending on the type and severity of the scarring. **Chemical peels**, **microdermabrasion**, and **laser resurfacing** are commonly used to improve skin texture and reduce the appearance of scars.

Microneedling and **radiofrequency treatments** are also effective in stimulating collagen production and smoothing out the skin.

For PIH, topical treatments containing ingredients like **vitamin C, niacinamide, azelaic acid**, and **retinoids** can help lighten dark spots and even out skin tone. Sun protection is crucial in preventing the darkening of PIH and protecting the skin from further damage. Using a broad-spectrum sunscreen with at least SPF 30 daily can help prevent worsening pigmentation and support the skin's healing process.

Managing acne requires a comprehensive approach that includes understanding the underlying causes, selecting appropriate treatments, and adopting healthy skincare and lifestyle practices. With the right combination of topical and oral treatments, along with supportive care and lifestyle adjustments, it is possible to achieve clearer skin and reduce the impact of acne on one's life.

4.2 Skin Aging: Prevention and Care

Skin aging is a natural process influenced by both intrinsic factors, such as genetics and the passage of time, and extrinsic factors, including sun exposure, pollution, and lifestyle choices. As we age, the skin undergoes several changes that affect its appearance and texture. The production of collagen and elastin, two proteins that provide structure and elasticity, decreases, leading to the formation of fine lines, wrinkles, and sagging. Additionally, the skin's natural renewal process slows down, resulting in a duller complexion and uneven skin tone. Effective anti-aging strategies focus on prevention, maintenance, and treatment to reduce the visible signs of aging and improve overall skin health.

Prevention is the cornerstone of any anti-aging strategy. The most effective way to prevent premature aging is to protect the skin from sun damage, which is responsible for up to 80% of visible aging signs. Ultraviolet (UV) radiation from the sun breaks down collagen and elastin fibers in the skin, leading to wrinkles, loss of firmness, and the development of age spots. Incorporating broad-spectrum sunscreen with at least SPF 30 into your daily skincare routine is essential to protect against both UVA and UVB rays. Applying sunscreen generously and reapplying every two hours when outdoors is critical to maintaining protection. Additionally, wearing protective clothing, such as wide-brimmed hats and UV-blocking sunglasses, can further reduce sun exposure.

Antioxidants play a significant role in preventing and mitigating the effects of aging by neutralizing free radicals that damage skin cells and accelerate aging. Free radicals are unstable molecules generated by exposure to UV radiation, pollution, and other environmental stressors. Antioxidants, such as vitamin C, vitamin E, and ferulic acid, help protect the skin from oxidative stress and enhance the skin's natural defense mechanisms. Incorporating antioxidant serums into your morning routine can provide a protective shield against daily environmental aggressors and boost the efficacy of sunscreen.

Retinoids are among the most effective treatments for reducing the visible signs of aging. Derived from vitamin A, retinoids, including retinol, tretinoin, and adapalene, promote cellular turnover, increase collagen production, and reduce the appearance of fine lines, wrinkles, and uneven skin tone. Retinoids work by accelerating the shedding of dead skin cells and stimulating the production of new cells, resulting in smoother, more youthful-looking skin. They also help fade age spots and improve skin texture by promoting the formation of new blood vessels. Because retinoids can cause irritation, especially when first introduced, it is advisable to start with a lower concentration and gradually increase it as the skin builds tolerance. Applying retinoids at night and following up with a moisturizer can help minimize dryness and peeling.

Peptides are another powerful ingredient in anti-aging skincare. Peptides are short chains of amino acids that serve as building blocks for proteins such as collagen and elastin. As we age, the natural production of these proteins decreases, leading to sagging skin and the formation of wrinkles. Topical peptides help stimulate collagen synthesis, improve skin elasticity, and reduce the appearance of fine lines and wrinkles. Peptide-rich serums and creams can be used daily to support the skin's structural integrity and enhance its resilience.

Hyaluronic acid is a hydrating powerhouse that helps plump the skin and reduce the appearance of fine lines. Naturally present in the skin, hyaluronic acid attracts and retains moisture, making it a valuable ingredient for maintaining skin hydration and elasticity. As we age, the skin's ability to retain moisture diminishes, leading to dryness and a loss of volume. Hyaluronic acid-based serums and creams help replenish moisture levels and create a smoother, more supple appearance. Products with different molecular weights of hyaluronic acid can penetrate various layers of the skin, providing both surface hydration and deeper moisture retention.

Exfoliation is a key component of an anti-aging routine, as it helps remove dead skin cells that can accumulate on the skin's surface, leading to a dull complexion and uneven texture. Regular exfoliation promotes cell turnover and enhances the absorption of other skincare products. There are two main types of exfoliation: chemical and physical. Chemical exfoliants, such as alpha hydroxy acids (AHAs) like glycolic acid and lactic acid, dissolve the bonds between dead skin cells, allowing them to be easily removed. AHAs also stimulate collagen production and improve skin texture. Physical exfoliants, such as scrubs or brushes, manually remove dead skin cells through friction. However, they should be used with caution to avoid over-exfoliation, which can damage the skin barrier and lead to irritation.

For those seeking more advanced anti-aging treatments, several in-office procedures can provide significant improvements in skin texture, tone, and firmness. **Chemical peels** involve the application of a chemical solution to exfoliate the skin's outer layers, revealing smoother, more even-toned skin beneath. Peels can vary in strength, from superficial to deep, depending on the desired results and downtime. Superficial peels use mild acids, such as glycolic or lactic acid, to provide gentle exfoliation, while medium and deep peels use stronger acids, such as trichloroacetic acid (TCA), to target deeper wrinkles and pigmentation.

Microdermabrasion is a non-invasive procedure that uses fine crystals or a diamond-tipped wand to exfoliate the outermost layer of the skin. This treatment helps improve the appearance of fine lines, age spots, and mild scarring by promoting cell turnover and collagen production. Microdermabrasion is suitable for all skin types and requires little to no downtime, making it a popular option for those seeking a quick refresh.

Microneedling is another effective anti-aging treatment that involves creating controlled micro-injuries in the skin using fine needles. This process stimulates the skin's natural wound-healing response, promoting the production of collagen and elastin. Microneedling is particularly effective for improving skin texture, reducing the appearance of fine lines, and minimizing scars. When combined with serums containing growth factors or peptides, microneedling can enhance the penetration and effectiveness of active ingredients.

Laser resurfacing is a more intensive treatment that uses focused beams of light to remove the outer layers of damaged skin and stimulate the growth of new, healthy skin. There are two main types of laser resurfacing: ablative and non-ablative. Ablative lasers remove the top layers of skin, providing more dramatic results for deeper wrinkles and scars but requiring a longer recovery period. Non-ablative lasers target deeper layers of the skin without removing the top layer, promoting collagen production and tightening the skin with minimal downtime. Laser resurfacing can be highly effective for reducing the appearance of wrinkles, age spots, and other signs of aging.

Radiofrequency (RF) treatments are non-invasive procedures that use radiofrequency energy to heat the deeper layers of the skin, stimulating collagen production and tightening sagging skin. RF treatments can be used on the face, neck, and body to improve skin laxity and reduce the appearance of wrinkles and fine lines. The results are gradual and improve over time as the skin produces more collagen. RF treatments are often combined with other modalities, such as microneedling or ultrasound, for enhanced results.

Injectable treatments, such as **botulinum toxin (Botox)** and **dermal fillers**, are popular options for addressing specific signs of aging. Botox is a neurotoxin that temporarily relaxes the muscles responsible for expression lines, such as frown lines, crow's feet, and forehead wrinkles. By preventing muscle contractions, Botox helps smooth out dynamic wrinkles and creates a more youthful appearance. Dermal fillers, on the other hand, are injectable gels made from substances like hyaluronic acid, calcium hydroxylapatite, or poly-L-lactic acid. Fillers are used to restore lost volume, smooth out deeper wrinkles, and enhance facial contours. They can also be used to plump the lips and improve the appearance of under-eye hollows. Both Botox and fillers provide immediate results with minimal downtime, making them popular choices for those seeking non-surgical anti-aging solutions.

In addition to these treatments, adopting a healthy lifestyle can significantly impact the aging process. Eating a balanced diet rich in antioxidants, vitamins, and minerals supports skin health and promotes a youthful appearance. Foods high in vitamin C, such as citrus fruits, berries, and leafy greens, help boost collagen production, while omega-3 fatty acids found in fish, nuts, and seeds provide anti-inflammatory benefits and support the skin's lipid barrier. Staying hydrated by drinking plenty of water helps maintain skin elasticity and plumpness.

Regular exercise improves blood circulation, delivering oxygen and nutrients to the skin and promoting a healthy glow. Additionally, exercise helps reduce stress, which can negatively affect the skin and accelerate aging. Incorporating stress management techniques, such as meditation, yoga, or deep breathing exercises, can help maintain hormonal balance and reduce the impact of stress on the skin.

Sleep is another crucial factor in the aging process. During sleep, the body undergoes repair and regeneration, including the production of collagen and elastin. Poor sleep quality can lead to increased stress levels, impaired skin barrier function, and a dull complexion. Prioritizing good sleep hygiene, such as maintaining a consistent sleep schedule, creating a relaxing bedtime routine, and ensuring a comfortable sleep environment, can support skin health and reduce the visible signs of aging.

By combining preventive measures with targeted treatments and a healthy lifestyle, it is possible to manage and reduce the signs of skin aging effectively. Whether through daily skincare routines, in-office procedures, or lifestyle adjustments, taking a proactive approach to anti-aging can help maintain a youthful, radiant complexion and support overall skin health.

4.3 Hyperpigmentation: Lightening Dark Spots

Hyperpigmentation is a common skin concern that manifests as darkened areas on the skin due to an excess production of melanin, the pigment responsible for skin color. These dark spots or patches can appear anywhere on the body and are often the result of sun exposure, hormonal changes, inflammation, or certain medications. Understanding the underlying causes of hyperpigmentation and exploring effective treatment options are crucial steps in achieving a more even skin tone and restoring a radiant complexion.

Hyperpigmentation can be caused by several factors, each contributing to the overproduction of melanin in different ways. One of the most common causes is **sun exposure**, which triggers the skin's natural defense mechanism to protect itself from UV radiation. When exposed to the sun, melanocytes—the cells responsible for producing melanin—become more active, leading to the development of sunspots or solar lentigines. These dark spots are typically found on areas of the skin that receive the most sun exposure, such as the face, hands, shoulders, and arms.

Hormonal changes are another significant cause of hyperpigmentation, particularly in women. Melasma, also known as "the mask of pregnancy," is a form of hyperpigmentation that occurs due to hormonal fluctuations, often during pregnancy, oral contraceptive use, or hormone replacement therapy. Melasma typically appears as brown or grayish-brown patches on the cheeks, forehead, nose, and upper lip. Unlike sunspots, melasma is more challenging to treat due to its hormonal origins and may require a combination of therapies to achieve noticeable results.

Post-inflammatory hyperpigmentation (PIH) occurs after an injury or inflammation to the skin, such as acne, eczema, or psoriasis. When the skin heals from inflammation, it can produce excess melanin, resulting in dark spots or patches. PIH is particularly common in individuals with darker skin tones, where melanocytes are more reactive to inflammation. PIH can also develop after cosmetic procedures like chemical peels, laser treatments, or dermabrasion if proper post-care is not followed.

Medications and certain medical conditions can also contribute to hyperpigmentation. Some medications, such as non-steroidal anti-inflammatory drugs (NSAIDs), tetracyclines, antimalarials, and certain chemotherapy drugs, can cause hyperpigmentation as a side effect. Additionally, conditions like Addison's disease and hemochromatosis can affect melanin production and lead to darkening of the skin.

Treating hyperpigmentation involves a multi-pronged approach that targets melanin production, promotes skin cell turnover, and protects the skin from further damage. One of the most effective ways to lighten dark spots is through the use of **topical treatments** that contain ingredients known to inhibit tyrosinase, the enzyme responsible for melanin production. **Hydroquinone** is one of the most potent tyrosinase inhibitors and has been used for decades to treat hyperpigmentation. It works by decreasing the production of melanin and breaking down existing melanin in the skin. Hydroquinone is typically prescribed at concentrations of 2% to 4% and should be used under the guidance of a healthcare provider due to its potential for irritation and side effects.

Vitamin C is a powerful antioxidant that also acts as a skin-brightening agent by inhibiting melanin production and neutralizing free radicals that can cause further pigmentation. Vitamin C serums are widely available and can be used daily to help lighten dark spots and improve overall skin tone. For best results, vitamin C should be applied in the morning before sunscreen to enhance its protective effects against UV radiation.

Niacinamide, also known as vitamin B3, is another effective ingredient for treating hyperpigmentation. Niacinamide works by inhibiting the transfer of melanin to the surface of the skin, thereby preventing the formation of new dark spots. It also has anti-inflammatory properties that can help reduce redness and irritation associated with PIH. Niacinamide is well-tolerated by most skin types and can be used in conjunction with other treatments to enhance its effectiveness.

Azelaic acid is a naturally occurring acid found in grains like barley, wheat, and rye. It has both exfoliating and skin-lightening properties, making it effective for treating PIH and melasma. Azelaic acid works by inhibiting tyrosinase activity and reducing the production of abnormal pigmentation. It is also beneficial for treating acne, as it helps to keep pores clear and reduce inflammation. Azelaic acid is available in over-the-counter formulations at 10% concentration and in prescription-strength formulations up to 20%.

Kojic acid is another tyrosinase inhibitor derived from fungi, such as Aspergillus and Penicillium species. Kojic acid not only helps to lighten dark spots but also provides antioxidant benefits that protect the skin from environmental damage. It is often used in combination with other brightening agents to enhance its effectiveness. However, kojic acid can be irritating to some individuals, especially when used at higher concentrations, so it should be introduced gradually into a skincare routine.

Chemical peels are an effective treatment option for hyperpigmentation, particularly for individuals with sunspots, melasma, or PIH. Chemical peels involve applying a solution of acids—such as glycolic acid, lactic acid, or trichloroacetic acid (TCA)—to the skin to exfoliate the outer layer and promote the regeneration of new, even-toned skin. The depth of the peel can vary from superficial to deep, depending on the severity of the hyperpigmentation and the desired results. Superficial peels provide mild exfoliation and require minimal downtime, while deeper peels offer more dramatic results but may require a longer recovery period.

Laser treatments are another advanced option for treating hyperpigmentation. Lasers work by targeting the melanin in the skin, breaking up the pigment, and allowing the body to gradually eliminate it. There are various types of lasers used for hyperpigmentation, including **fractional lasers**, **intense pulsed light (IPL)**, and **Q-switched lasers**. Fractional lasers are effective for treating sunspots and PIH, while Q-switched lasers are often used for deeper pigmentation, such as melasma. Laser treatments should be performed by a qualified professional, as improper use can lead to further pigmentation or scarring.

Microneedling, also known as collagen induction therapy, is a minimally invasive procedure that involves using fine needles to create micro-injuries in the skin. These micro-injuries stimulate the skin's natural healing process, promoting collagen production and improving the appearance of hyperpigmentation. Microneedling can be combined with topical treatments, such as vitamin C or kojic acid, to enhance their penetration and effectiveness. This treatment is suitable for various skin types and can help improve the overall texture and tone of the skin.

Cryotherapy is a treatment that involves using liquid nitrogen to freeze and destroy hyperpigmented cells. It is most commonly used for treating sunspots or age spots and is generally performed in a clinical setting. While effective, cryotherapy can cause temporary redness, swelling, and, in some cases, blistering or scabbing as the treated area heals.

In addition to these treatments, maintaining a consistent skincare routine that includes **daily sun protection** is crucial for managing hyperpigmentation and preventing further darkening. Sun exposure can exacerbate existing pigmentation and trigger the formation of new spots, so applying a broad-spectrum sunscreen with at least SPF 30 every day is essential. Reapplying sunscreen every two hours when outdoors, wearing protective clothing, and seeking shade during peak sun hours can further reduce the risk of sun-induced pigmentation.

Proper skincare also involves regular exfoliation to remove dead skin cells and promote cell turnover. Gentle exfoliation with products containing AHAs or BHAs can help improve the appearance of hyperpigmentation by accelerating the removal of pigmented cells and enhancing the absorption of brightening agents. However, it is important to avoid over-exfoliating, as this can irritate the skin and worsen hyperpigmentation.

For those dealing with melasma or stubborn pigmentation, it may be necessary to combine multiple treatment modalities to achieve the best results. Consulting with a dermatologist or skincare professional can help determine the most appropriate treatment plan based on the specific type and severity of hyperpigmentation. With a combination of targeted treatments, protective measures, and consistent skincare, it is possible to reduce the appearance of dark spots and achieve a more even, radiant complexion.

4.4 Sensitivity and Rosacea: How to Manage Them

Sensitive skin and rosacea are common concerns that can cause significant discomfort and affect one's confidence. Sensitive skin is characterized by a heightened response to external stimuli, such as skincare products, environmental factors, or changes in weather, leading to redness, itching, stinging, or burning sensations. Rosacea is a chronic skin condition that primarily affects the face, causing redness, visible blood vessels, and, in some cases, acne-like breakouts. While sensitive skin and rosacea are distinct conditions, they often overlap, requiring a gentle, targeted approach to management and care. Understanding the triggers and selecting appropriate products and habits are key to reducing irritation and maintaining a healthy, calm complexion.

Sensitive skin can result from a weakened skin barrier, which is less effective at protecting against environmental aggressors and retaining moisture. This can lead to increased transepidermal water loss (TEWL), making the skin more prone to dryness and irritation. Common triggers for sensitive skin include harsh skincare ingredients, such as fragrances, alcohol, and certain preservatives, as well as environmental factors like extreme temperatures, wind, and pollution. Stress, hormonal changes, and even diet can also exacerbate sensitivity.

Rosacea, on the other hand, is a chronic inflammatory condition that primarily affects individuals with fair skin, although it can occur in any skin type. The exact cause of rosacea is not fully understood, but it is believed to involve a combination of genetic, environmental, and vascular factors. Triggers for rosacea flare-ups can include sun exposure, hot or spicy foods, alcohol, extreme temperatures, stress, and certain skincare products. Rosacea often presents as persistent redness on the cheeks, nose, chin, and forehead, with visible blood vessels and, in some cases, pustules that resemble acne. Unlike acne, however, rosacea does not typically produce blackheads or whiteheads.

To effectively manage sensitive skin and rosacea, it is important to adopt a gentle skincare routine that focuses on soothing and strengthening the skin barrier. The following steps outline a comprehensive approach to caring for sensitive and rosacea-prone skin:

1. **Choose a Gentle Cleanser**: Cleansing is a crucial step in any skincare routine, but for sensitive or rosacea-prone skin, it is important to use a gentle, non-foaming cleanser that does not strip the skin of its natural oils. Look for cleansers that are free from sulfates, fragrances, and alcohol, which can irritate the skin and exacerbate sensitivity. Ingredients like glycerin, allantoin, and chamomile extract are soothing and help to maintain the skin's natural moisture balance. Cleansing should be done with lukewarm water, as hot water can further irritate sensitive skin and trigger rosacea flare-ups.

2. **Incorporate Soothing Ingredients**: Calming ingredients that help reduce redness and irritation are essential for managing sensitive skin and rosacea. Niacinamide, also known as vitamin B3, is a versatile ingredient that helps strengthen the skin barrier, reduce inflammation, and improve overall skin tone. It is well-tolerated by most skin types and can be used in conjunction with other soothing ingredients like panthenol (provitamin B5), which helps to hydrate and repair the skin. Azelaic acid is another beneficial ingredient for rosacea, as it has anti-inflammatory and

anti-bacterial properties that can help reduce redness and prevent pustules without causing irritation.

3. **Moisturize Regularly**: Keeping the skin well-moisturized is vital for maintaining a healthy skin barrier and reducing sensitivity. Choose a moisturizer that is free from potential irritants, such as fragrances, dyes, and harsh preservatives. Look for formulations that contain ceramides, fatty acids, and hyaluronic acid to help reinforce the skin barrier and lock in moisture. A lightweight, non-greasy moisturizer can provide sufficient hydration without clogging pores or feeling heavy on the skin. For those with rosacea, a moisturizer that includes green tea extract or feverfew can help soothe redness and calm the skin.

4. **Protect the Skin from the Sun**: Sun exposure is a common trigger for both sensitive skin and rosacea, making sun protection a priority. Use a broad-spectrum sunscreen with at least SPF 30 daily, even on cloudy days or when indoors, as UV rays can penetrate windows. Mineral sunscreens containing zinc oxide or titanium dioxide are often better tolerated by sensitive skin and provide effective protection without causing irritation. To further protect against sun damage, wear protective clothing, such as wide-brimmed hats and UV-blocking sunglasses, and seek shade during peak sun hours.

5. **Avoid Known Triggers**: Identifying and avoiding triggers is key to managing sensitivity and rosacea. Keep a skincare diary to track potential triggers, such as specific products, foods, or environmental conditions that cause flare-ups. Common triggers for rosacea include spicy foods, hot drinks, alcohol, and extreme temperatures. For sensitive skin, harsh skincare ingredients, over-exfoliation, and strong fragrances are frequent culprits. By identifying these triggers, you can make more informed choices about your skincare and lifestyle habits.

6. **Use Targeted Treatments for Rosacea**: For individuals with rosacea, topical treatments that reduce redness and inflammation can be beneficial. Metronidazole, azelaic acid, and ivermectin are commonly prescribed topical medications that help reduce the symptoms of rosacea. These treatments work by reducing inflammation and the presence of Demodex mites, which are believed to play a role in some cases of rosacea. It is important to use these medications as directed by a healthcare provider and to be patient, as results may take several weeks to become noticeable.

7. **Consider Laser and Light-Based Therapies**: For more severe cases of rosacea, laser and light-based therapies can offer effective solutions. Intense pulsed

light (IPL) therapy targets blood vessels beneath the skin's surface, reducing redness and flushing associated with rosacea. Vascular lasers, such as the pulsed dye laser (PDL), can also target and shrink visible blood vessels, leading to a more even skin tone. These treatments should be performed by a qualified dermatologist or skincare professional and may require multiple sessions for optimal results.

8. **Maintain a Simple, Consistent Routine**: Keeping your skincare routine simple and consistent is key to managing sensitive skin and rosacea. Avoid overloading the skin with too many products, which can increase the risk of irritation and worsen symptoms. Stick to a basic routine that includes a gentle cleanser, a soothing moisturizer, and sun protection. Introduce new products slowly, one at a time, and perform patch tests to assess how your skin reacts. Consistency is crucial in building a resilient skin barrier and reducing sensitivity over time.

9. **Adopt Healthy Lifestyle Habits**: Lifestyle choices can significantly impact skin sensitivity and rosacea. Stress management techniques, such as meditation, yoga, or deep breathing exercises, can help reduce flare-ups triggered by emotional stress. Maintaining a balanced diet rich in anti-inflammatory foods, such as fruits, vegetables, omega-3 fatty acids, and whole grains, can

also support skin health. Reducing alcohol and caffeine intake may be beneficial for some individuals, as these substances can exacerbate rosacea symptoms.

10. **Consult with a Dermatologist**: If you have persistent sensitivity or rosacea that does not improve with over-the-counter products and lifestyle changes, consult with a dermatologist. A healthcare professional can provide a personalized treatment plan tailored to your specific skin needs and recommend prescription medications or in-office treatments if necessary. Early intervention and proper management can help control symptoms and prevent further skin damage.

Managing sensitive skin and rosacea requires a thoughtful and consistent approach to skincare and lifestyle. By understanding the triggers, choosing gentle and soothing products, and adopting healthy habits, it is possible to reduce irritation, improve skin resilience, and achieve a calmer, healthier complexion.

CHAPTER 5: SKINCARE IN THE CONTEXT OF A HEALTHY LIFESTYLE

5.1 Nutrition and Skin

The connection between nutrition and skin health is profound and multifaceted. What we eat not only affects our overall health but also has a significant impact on our skin's appearance and function. The skin is the body's largest organ, and like any other organ, it relies on essential nutrients to function optimally. A balanced diet rich in vitamins, minerals, antioxidants, and other key nutrients can help maintain the skin's integrity, support its natural repair mechanisms, and protect it from environmental damage. Understanding the role of nutrition in skincare can empower individuals to make dietary choices that enhance their skin health and contribute to a more radiant, youthful complexion.

One of the most critical nutrients for skin health is **vitamin C**, a powerful antioxidant that plays a crucial role in collagen synthesis. Collagen is a structural protein that provides strength and elasticity to the skin. As we age, collagen production naturally decreases, leading to the formation of wrinkles and sagging skin. Vitamin C helps to stimulate collagen production, maintain the skin's firmness, and protect against oxidative damage caused by free radicals. Incorporating foods rich in vitamin C, such as citrus fruits, strawberries, bell peppers, broccoli, and kiwi, into your diet can help support collagen production and enhance skin's resilience.

Vitamin E is another essential antioxidant that protects the skin from oxidative stress and environmental damage, such as UV radiation and pollution. It works by neutralizing free radicals and preventing lipid peroxidation, which can damage the skin's barrier and lead to inflammation and premature aging. Foods high in vitamin E, such as almonds, sunflower seeds, spinach, and avocados, can help maintain the skin's moisture barrier and improve its ability to retain hydration. Vitamin E also has anti-inflammatory properties, which can be particularly beneficial for individuals with sensitive or reactive skin.

Vitamin A and its derivatives, such as retinoids, are well-known for their role in skin health. Vitamin A is essential for maintaining the integrity of the skin's epithelial tissues, promoting cell turnover, and supporting the skin's natural repair processes. Retinoids, derived from vitamin A, are widely used in skincare products to treat acne, reduce hyperpigmentation, and minimize fine lines and wrinkles. Including foods rich in beta-carotene, a precursor to vitamin A, such as carrots, sweet potatoes, spinach, and kale, can provide the skin with the necessary nutrients to maintain its health and vitality.

Zinc is a mineral that plays a vital role in skin health, particularly in wound healing and inflammation control. Zinc is involved in various enzymatic reactions that regulate cell growth, repair damaged tissues, and protect against UV radiation. It also has antibacterial properties that can help prevent acne by reducing the growth of *Propionibacterium acnes*, the bacteria that contributes to acne development. Foods rich in zinc, such as oysters, red meat, poultry, beans, nuts, and seeds, can support the skin's immune function and help maintain a clear, healthy complexion.

Omega-3 fatty acids are essential fats that have anti-inflammatory properties and are critical for maintaining the skin's lipid barrier. A strong lipid barrier helps retain moisture, prevent dryness, and protect the skin from environmental aggressors. Omega-3 fatty acids, particularly eicosapentaenoic acid (EPA) and docosahexaenoic acid (DHA), can help reduce inflammation in the skin, making them beneficial for individuals with inflammatory skin conditions such as eczema, psoriasis, and acne. Foods rich in omega-3s, such as fatty fish (salmon, mackerel, sardines), flaxseeds, chia seeds, and walnuts, can help keep the skin supple, hydrated, and less prone to irritation.

Biotin, also known as vitamin B7, is another nutrient crucial for skin health. Biotin plays a role in the maintenance of healthy skin by supporting the production of fatty acids and promoting the health of the skin barrier. While biotin deficiency is rare, ensuring an adequate intake through foods like eggs, nuts, seeds, and whole grains can help maintain healthy skin, hair, and nails.

Selenium is a trace mineral that works as a powerful antioxidant, protecting the skin from free radical damage and supporting its natural defense mechanisms. Selenium is also involved in DNA repair and helps reduce inflammation, making it beneficial for overall skin health and resilience. Foods high in selenium, such as Brazil nuts, tuna, eggs, and whole grains, can provide the skin with the nutrients it needs to maintain its integrity and appearance.

Hydration is another critical aspect of nutrition that affects skin health. Proper hydration is essential for maintaining the skin's moisture balance and elasticity. Drinking adequate water throughout the day helps flush out toxins, supports skin metabolism, and keeps the skin plump and hydrated. Dehydration can lead to dryness, dullness, and increased visibility of fine lines and wrinkles. In addition to drinking water, consuming water-rich foods such as cucumbers, watermelon, oranges, and lettuce can contribute to overall hydration and promote a healthy, glowing complexion.

Probiotics and gut health are also gaining recognition for their role in skin health. A healthy gut microbiome supports overall immune function and can help reduce inflammation throughout the body, including the skin. Probiotics, found in fermented foods like yogurt, kefir, sauerkraut, kimchi, and kombucha, help maintain a balanced gut microbiota, which in turn can positively impact skin conditions such as acne, eczema, and rosacea. Incorporating probiotic-rich foods into your diet can support gut health and contribute to a clearer, healthier complexion.

A diet high in **antioxidant-rich foods** can provide additional protection against environmental damage and premature aging. Antioxidants help neutralize free radicals, which are unstable molecules generated by exposure to UV radiation, pollution, and other environmental stressors. Foods rich in antioxidants, such as berries (blueberries, raspberries, strawberries), dark leafy greens, nuts, and dark chocolate, can help protect the skin from oxidative stress and maintain its youthful appearance.

While nutrition plays a vital role in skin health, it is also important to recognize the impact of certain foods that can negatively affect the skin. Diets high in refined sugars, processed foods, and dairy have been associated with an increased risk of acne and other skin conditions. Excessive consumption of sugar and high-glycemic-index foods can lead to spikes in blood sugar levels, triggering an inflammatory response and increasing sebum production. This can contribute to clogged pores and acne breakouts. Similarly, some studies suggest that dairy products, particularly skim milk, may exacerbate acne due to hormones and bioactive molecules present in milk. Reducing the intake of these foods and focusing on a balanced diet rich in whole, unprocessed foods can help improve skin health and reduce the risk of flare-ups.

In addition to specific nutrients, maintaining a balanced and varied diet that includes a wide range of fruits, vegetables, lean proteins, healthy fats, and whole grains is essential for overall skin health. A well-rounded diet ensures that the skin receives a broad spectrum of vitamins, minerals, and antioxidants necessary for maintaining its integrity, function, and appearance. By making conscious dietary choices that prioritize nutrient-dense foods, individuals can support their skin's health from within and enhance the effectiveness of their skincare routines.

Understanding the relationship between nutrition and skin health is crucial for achieving a radiant, youthful complexion. By incorporating essential nutrients and making mindful dietary choices, you can nourish your skin from the inside out, supporting its natural ability to heal, renew, and protect itself against environmental damage.

5.2 Managing Stress and Its Impact on Skin

Stress is an inevitable part of life, but its impact on the skin is often underestimated. Chronic stress can wreak havoc on skin health, exacerbating existing conditions and triggering new problems. The skin, being the body's largest organ, is highly sensitive to emotional and physiological changes. When stress becomes chronic, it can lead to a range of skin issues, including acne, eczema, psoriasis, rosacea, and premature aging. Understanding the connection between stress and skin health and implementing strategies to manage stress effectively can help improve skin condition and overall well-being.

The skin and the nervous system are intimately connected through a complex network known as the **psychoneuroimmunological pathway**. This connection means that emotional and psychological states can directly influence skin health. When the body experiences stress, it triggers the release of stress hormones, such as cortisol and adrenaline, which activate the body's "fight or flight" response. While this response is essential for short-term survival, prolonged exposure to elevated stress hormones can negatively affect the skin.

Cortisol, the primary stress hormone, has several detrimental effects on the skin when present in high levels over an extended period. Cortisol increases sebum production, leading to oily skin and clogged pores, which can exacerbate acne. It also impairs the skin's barrier function, reducing its ability to retain moisture and protect against external aggressors. This compromised barrier can result in dryness, irritation, and increased sensitivity, making the skin more susceptible to environmental damage and infections.

Stress also promotes **inflammation**, which can trigger or worsen inflammatory skin conditions such as eczema, psoriasis, and rosacea. For individuals with these conditions, stress can lead to flare-ups, characterized by redness, itching, and discomfort. The inflammatory response is partly due to the release of neuropeptides and pro-inflammatory cytokines, which stimulate the immune system and cause inflammation in the skin. Over time, chronic inflammation can damage skin cells, accelerate aging, and impair the skin's natural repair processes.

Additionally, stress can affect the skin's ability to heal and regenerate. Studies have shown that stressed skin has a slower wound healing process due to impaired cell turnover and reduced collagen production. Collagen is essential for maintaining skin elasticity and firmness, and its depletion can lead to the formation of fine lines, wrinkles, and sagging. Furthermore, stress can disrupt sleep patterns, leading to poor sleep quality. During sleep, the body undergoes repair and regeneration, including the production of collagen and other essential proteins. Lack of sleep can result in dull, tired-looking skin and exacerbate the appearance of dark circles and puffiness.

Given the profound impact of stress on skin health, it is essential to adopt strategies to manage stress effectively. Here are some evidence-based approaches to reducing stress and improving skin condition:

1. **Mindfulness and Meditation**: Mindfulness practices, such as meditation and deep breathing exercises, can help reduce stress by promoting relaxation and emotional regulation. Mindfulness involves paying attention to the present moment and accepting it without judgment, which can help calm the mind and reduce the physiological effects of stress. Studies have shown that regular meditation can lower cortisol levels, reduce inflammation, and improve overall skin health. Incorporating just a few minutes of mindfulness practice into your daily routine can have a significant impact on stress levels and skin condition.

2. **Physical Exercise**: Regular physical activity is a powerful stress-relief tool that also benefits the skin. Exercise promotes the release of endorphins, known as "feel-good" hormones, which help improve mood and reduce stress. It also enhances blood circulation, delivering oxygen and nutrients to the skin and promoting a healthy glow. Exercise can also support the body's detoxification processes, helping to remove toxins that can contribute to skin problems. Aim for at least 30 minutes of moderate exercise most days of the week, whether it's brisk walking, jogging, yoga, or dancing, to reap the skin and stress-reducing benefits.

3. **Balanced Nutrition**: A diet rich in antioxidants, vitamins, and minerals can help combat the effects of stress on the skin. Certain foods, such as berries, leafy greens, nuts, seeds, and fish, contain nutrients that support skin health and reduce inflammation. Omega-3 fatty acids, found in fatty fish like salmon and mackerel, have anti-inflammatory properties that can help soothe stressed skin. Avoiding high-glycemic foods and refined sugars can prevent spikes in blood sugar and insulin levels, which can exacerbate acne and other skin conditions. Staying hydrated by drinking plenty of water throughout the day is also essential for maintaining skin hydration and function.

4. **Adequate Sleep**: Quality sleep is vital for skin health, as it allows the body to repair and regenerate. During deep sleep, the body produces collagen and other essential proteins that maintain skin elasticity and firmness. Aim for 7-9 hours of uninterrupted sleep per night to ensure optimal skin regeneration and recovery. Establishing a regular sleep routine, creating a calming bedtime environment, and avoiding screens and stimulants before bed can help improve sleep quality and reduce the impact of stress on the skin.

5. **Skincare Routine**: Maintaining a consistent skincare routine that includes gentle cleansing, moisturizing, and

sun protection is crucial for managing stress-related skin issues. Using skincare products with soothing and calming ingredients, such as aloe vera, chamomile, green tea, and niacinamide, can help reduce inflammation and protect the skin barrier. Avoiding harsh products that strip the skin of its natural oils or contain irritating ingredients can prevent further aggravation of sensitive or stressed skin. Incorporating regular facial massages or using a jade roller can also promote relaxation and improve blood circulation, enhancing the skin's natural glow.

6. **Social Support and Connection**: Building and maintaining strong social connections can provide emotional support and reduce stress. Talking to friends, family, or a therapist about stressors can help alleviate emotional burden and provide perspective. Engaging in social activities, volunteering, or joining a support group can foster a sense of belonging and reduce feelings of isolation, which can contribute to stress.

7. **Creative Outlets**: Engaging in creative activities, such as painting, writing, or playing a musical instrument, can serve as a therapeutic outlet for stress relief. Creative expression allows for emotional release and can provide a sense of accomplishment and joy. Finding a hobby or activity that brings you pleasure and relaxation can help

manage stress levels and improve overall well-being, positively impacting skin health.

8. **Professional Support**: If stress is overwhelming or persistent, seeking professional support from a therapist, counselor, or dermatologist can be beneficial. Cognitive-behavioral therapy (CBT) and other therapeutic approaches can help develop coping strategies and address the root causes of stress. Dermatologists can provide targeted treatments and recommendations for managing stress-related skin conditions, such as acne, eczema, or rosacea.

Managing stress is an ongoing process that requires a combination of self-care practices, lifestyle adjustments, and professional support when necessary. By understanding the link between stress and skin health and adopting effective stress-reduction strategies, individuals can improve their skin condition, enhance their overall well-being, and promote a healthier, more radiant complexion.

5.3 Sleep and Skin Regeneration

Sleep is a vital component of overall health and plays a crucial role in skin regeneration and repair. The phrase "beauty sleep" is more than just a saying; it reflects the essential function of sleep in maintaining skin health and appearance. During sleep, the body undergoes critical repair processes, including the renewal of skin cells, production of collagen, and healing of daily damage caused by environmental stressors. Poor sleep quality can negatively impact these processes, leading to a range of skin issues such as dullness, fine lines, dark circles, and even exacerbating conditions like acne and eczema. Understanding the relationship between sleep and skin health, and adopting strategies to improve sleep quality, can lead to a more radiant and youthful complexion.

The skin follows a natural circadian rhythm, a 24-hour cycle that regulates various biological processes, including cell regeneration and repair. During the day, the skin is primarily focused on protecting itself from environmental aggressors, such as UV radiation, pollution, and free radicals. At night, the skin shifts its focus to recovery and repair, when cell turnover is at its peak, and the production of essential proteins, such as collagen and elastin, is maximized. These proteins are critical for maintaining skin elasticity, firmness, and strength.

Collagen production is a key process that occurs during sleep. Collagen is a structural protein that gives the skin its strength and resilience. As we age, collagen production naturally declines, leading to the formation of wrinkles and sagging skin. Sleep stimulates collagen synthesis, helping to replenish and maintain the skin's structural integrity. Adequate sleep allows the body to produce sufficient collagen to repair damage caused by daily wear and tear, keeping the skin smooth and firm. A lack of sleep can impair collagen production, accelerating the aging process and contributing to the development of fine lines and wrinkles.

In addition to collagen production, sleep is essential for maintaining proper hydration and moisture balance in the skin. During the deep stages of sleep, the body's hydration levels are rebalanced, allowing the skin to recover moisture lost throughout the day. This process helps maintain the skin's natural barrier function, preventing transepidermal water loss (TEWL) and keeping the skin hydrated and plump. Poor sleep quality can disrupt this balance, leading to dryness, flakiness, and a compromised skin barrier that is more susceptible to irritation and inflammation.

Sleep also plays a crucial role in reducing inflammation, a key factor in many skin conditions such as acne, eczema, psoriasis, and rosacea. Chronic lack of sleep can lead to elevated levels of cortisol, the stress hormone, which can increase inflammation and exacerbate these conditions. By promoting adequate sleep, the body can regulate cortisol levels, reduce inflammation, and create a more favorable environment for skin healing and renewal.

Dark circles and puffiness under the eyes are common signs of sleep deprivation. The skin around the eyes is thin and delicate, making it more susceptible to fluid retention and blood vessel visibility. Lack of sleep can cause blood vessels to dilate, leading to dark circles, while fluid retention can result in puffiness or bags under the eyes. Adequate sleep helps reduce these signs of fatigue, allowing the skin around the eyes to appear brighter and more refreshed.

To maximize the benefits of sleep for skin health, it is essential to adopt practices that promote quality sleep. Here are some strategies to improve sleep and enhance skin regeneration:

1. **Establish a Consistent Sleep Schedule**: Going to bed and waking up at the same time every day helps regulate the body's internal clock and improves sleep quality. Consistency in sleep patterns reinforces the body's natural circadian rhythm, ensuring that the skin undergoes its repair and renewal processes effectively. Aim to get 7-9 hours of uninterrupted sleep each night to support optimal skin health.

2. **Create a Relaxing Bedtime Routine**: Establishing a calming pre-sleep routine can signal to the body that it is time to wind down and prepare for sleep. Activities such as reading a book, taking a warm bath, practicing gentle yoga, or engaging in mindfulness meditation can help reduce stress and promote relaxation. Avoid stimulating activities, such as watching television or using electronic devices, which emit blue light that can interfere with the production of melatonin, the sleep hormone.

3. **Optimize the Sleep Environment**: Creating a sleep-friendly environment is crucial for improving sleep quality. Ensure that the bedroom is dark, quiet, and cool, as these conditions promote better sleep. Consider using blackout curtains, earplugs, or white noise machines to minimize disruptions. Investing in a comfortable mattress and pillows can also support proper spinal alignment and improve sleep comfort.

4. **Limit Stimulants and Alcohol**: Caffeine and nicotine are stimulants that can interfere with sleep by increasing alertness and delaying the onset of sleep. Avoid consuming caffeinated beverages, such as coffee, tea, or energy drinks, in the afternoon or evening. Similarly, while alcohol may initially induce drowsiness, it can disrupt sleep cycles and reduce the quality of sleep. Limiting alcohol intake, especially close to bedtime, can help maintain a more restful sleep.

5. **Practice Good Sleep Hygiene**: Good sleep hygiene involves habits that promote healthy sleep patterns. This includes keeping the bedroom environment conducive to sleep, avoiding heavy meals or excessive fluid intake before bed, and managing stress through relaxation techniques. Additionally, engaging in regular physical activity can help improve sleep quality, but it is best to

avoid vigorous exercise close to bedtime, as it can increase alertness and delay sleep onset.

6. **Incorporate a Nighttime Skincare Routine**: Taking care of the skin before bed can enhance the benefits of sleep for skin health. A nighttime skincare routine that includes gentle cleansing, moisturizing, and applying targeted treatments can support the skin's natural repair processes. Using products with ingredients such as hyaluronic acid, retinoids, and peptides can help boost hydration, promote cell turnover, and stimulate collagen production. Ensuring that the skin is clean and well-moisturized before bed can also prevent clogged pores and reduce the risk of breakouts.

7. **Manage Stress Effectively**: Chronic stress can negatively impact sleep quality and skin health. Implementing stress-reduction techniques, such as mindfulness meditation, deep breathing exercises, or journaling, can help manage stress and promote relaxation. Reducing stress not only improves sleep quality but also supports overall skin health by minimizing inflammation and promoting a balanced hormonal environment.

8. **Stay Hydrated Throughout the Day**: Proper hydration is essential for skin health, and it also affects sleep quality. Dehydration can lead to dry mouth and

nasal passages, making it difficult to sleep comfortably. Drinking adequate water throughout the day helps maintain hydration levels, supporting both sleep quality and skin health. However, it is advisable to limit fluid intake in the hours leading up to bedtime to prevent frequent nighttime awakenings.

By prioritizing quality sleep and adopting healthy sleep habits, individuals can enhance the skin's natural repair and regeneration processes. Adequate sleep supports collagen production, reduces inflammation, and maintains proper hydration levels, all of which contribute to a more radiant and youthful complexion. Incorporating these practices into a daily routine can lead to improved skin health and a more refreshed, rejuvenated appearance.

CHAPTER 6: MYTHS AND TRUTHS IN SKINCARE

6.1 Demystifying Misconceptions

The world of skincare is rife with myths and misconceptions, often fueled by marketing claims, anecdotal advice, and outdated beliefs. These myths can lead to ineffective skincare practices, wasted resources, and, in some cases, harm to the skin. Demystifying these common misconceptions and understanding the truths based on scientific evidence can help individuals make more informed decisions about their skincare routines and achieve healthier, more radiant skin.

One of the most pervasive myths in skincare is that **natural ingredients are always better for the skin**. While natural ingredients like aloe vera, chamomile, and green tea can have soothing and antioxidant properties, not all natural substances are safe or effective for every skin type. For instance, essential oils, which are often touted for their natural benefits, can be irritating to sensitive skin and may cause allergic reactions or phototoxicity when exposed to sunlight. Conversely, some synthetic ingredients, such as hyaluronic acid and ceramides, are scientifically formulated to mimic or enhance the skin's natural components, providing targeted benefits without the risk of irritation. The effectiveness of a skincare ingredient depends on its formulation, concentration, and how it interacts with the skin, not simply whether it is natural or synthetic.

Another common misconception is that **drinking more water alone will hydrate the skin**. While staying hydrated is essential for overall health and can support skin function, drinking water alone does not directly hydrate the skin's outer layers. The skin's hydration levels are more closely related to the health of the skin barrier and the topical application of moisturizing products that contain humectants, emollients, and occlusives. Ingredients like hyaluronic acid, glycerin, and urea attract and retain moisture in the skin, while oils and butters form a protective layer to prevent water loss. To achieve optimal hydration, it is necessary to combine adequate water intake with a consistent skincare routine that includes moisturizers tailored to the skin type.

The belief that **oily skin does not need a moisturizer** is another widespread myth that can lead to suboptimal skincare practices. People with oily skin often skip moisturizers, fearing they will make their skin oilier or cause breakouts. However, all skin types, including oily and acne-prone skin, need hydration to maintain a healthy barrier function. When oily skin is dehydrated, it can overcompensate by producing even more oil, exacerbating the problem. Using a lightweight, non-comedogenic moisturizer can provide essential hydration without clogging pores or adding excess shine. Moisturizers formulated with ingredients like hyaluronic acid, niacinamide, and salicylic acid can help balance oil production while keeping the skin hydrated and clear.

The idea that **sunscreen is only necessary on sunny days** is a dangerous myth that can expose the skin to harmful UV radiation year-round. Ultraviolet (UV) rays are present even on cloudy days and can penetrate through windows, causing cumulative damage that leads to premature aging, hyperpigmentation, and an increased risk of skin cancer. UVA rays, in particular, are present throughout the year and can penetrate deeper into the skin, causing long-term damage to collagen and elastin fibers. Daily application of broad-spectrum sunscreen with at least SPF 30 is essential, regardless of weather conditions, to protect the skin from UV damage and maintain a healthy, youthful appearance.

Another common myth is that **expensive skincare products are always more effective** than their affordable counterparts. While luxury skincare brands often market their products as having superior ingredients or advanced formulations, the price of a product does not necessarily correlate with its efficacy. Many affordable skincare products contain the same active ingredients as high-end brands and can deliver comparable results. The effectiveness of a skincare product depends on the quality and concentration of its active ingredients, its formulation, and how well it suits an individual's skin type and concerns. It is important to evaluate products based on their ingredient list and clinical evidence rather than price alone.

The misconception that **acne is caused by poor hygiene** is another myth that can lead to over-cleansing and irritation. Acne is a multifactorial condition influenced by genetics, hormones, inflammation, and bacteria, not just dirt or surface oils. Over-cleansing or using harsh scrubs can strip the skin of its natural oils, leading to increased oil production and worsening acne. A gentle cleansing routine that removes excess oil and impurities without disrupting the skin barrier is key to managing acne. Ingredients like salicylic acid, benzoyl peroxide, and retinoids can help target acne-causing factors more effectively than excessive washing.

The notion that **pores can open and close** like doors is another widespread myth. Pores do not have muscles and cannot open or close. Their appearance can change due to factors such as oil production, clogged pores, and skin elasticity. When pores are clogged with excess oil, dead skin cells, or debris, they may appear larger. Treatments like exfoliation, chemical peels, and ingredients such as retinoids and salicylic acid can help clear pores and reduce their appearance by promoting skin turnover and removing buildup. Using products that help tighten and firm the skin, such as niacinamide and collagen-boosting peptides, can also minimize the appearance of enlarged pores.

The belief that **you must "feel the burn" for a product to be effective** is a misconception that can lead to skin damage. A tingling or burning sensation is often a sign of irritation, not effectiveness. While some active ingredients, like alpha hydroxy acids (AHAs) or retinoids, may cause mild tingling as the skin adjusts, a burning sensation indicates that the product is too harsh or is causing an adverse reaction. It is essential to choose products that suit your skin type and tolerance levels and to introduce potent actives gradually to avoid irritation and support the skin's health.

Lastly, the idea that **aging can be completely prevented with skincare** is misleading. While a consistent skincare routine with sun protection, hydration, and targeted treatments can significantly delay the signs of aging and improve the skin's appearance, aging is a natural process influenced by genetics, lifestyle, and environmental factors. Skincare can help manage and minimize visible signs of aging, such as fine lines, wrinkles, and age spots, but it cannot stop the aging process entirely. Embracing a holistic approach that includes healthy lifestyle choices, such as a balanced diet, regular exercise, stress management, and sufficient sleep, along with a well-formulated skincare routine, can help maintain a youthful, healthy complexion for as long as possible.

By debunking these common skincare myths and understanding the science behind skin health, individuals can make more informed choices and develop effective skincare routines tailored to their unique needs. This evidence-based approach can help achieve healthier, more radiant skin and avoid the pitfalls of misinformation and ineffective practices.

6.2 The Truth About Natural Ingredients

The skincare industry has seen a significant rise in the popularity of natural ingredients, driven by a growing consumer desire for clean, safe, and effective products. However, not all natural ingredients are created equal, and the term "natural" itself is often used as a marketing strategy rather than an indicator of efficacy or safety. Understanding the science behind natural ingredients and distinguishing between those that are genuinely beneficial and those that are more hype than help is crucial for making informed skincare choices.

One of the most celebrated natural ingredients in skincare is **aloe vera.** Known for its soothing and hydrating properties, aloe vera has been used for centuries to treat burns, wounds, and skin irritation. The clear gel from the aloe vera plant contains vitamins, minerals, enzymes, and amino acids that help to calm inflammation and promote skin healing. Its lightweight, water-rich composition makes it an excellent hydrator for all skin types, particularly for soothing sunburns or sensitive skin. Scientific studies have supported aloe vera's ability to accelerate wound healing and reduce redness, validating its effectiveness beyond marketing claims.

Green tea extract is another natural ingredient with a strong scientific backing. Rich in polyphenols, particularly epigallocatechin gallate (EGCG), green tea extract has potent antioxidant and anti-inflammatory properties. It helps protect the skin from UV damage, reduce redness and irritation, and improve skin elasticity. Green tea's ability to neutralize free radicals makes it a valuable addition to skincare formulations aimed at preventing premature aging and protecting against environmental stressors. Clinical research has demonstrated green tea's effectiveness in reducing acne and soothing rosacea, proving it to be more than just a marketing trend.

Chamomile is widely recognized for its calming and anti-inflammatory properties. Containing compounds like bisabolol and chamazulene, chamomile extract helps soothe irritated skin, reduce redness, and promote healing. It is often found in products designed for sensitive skin or those suffering from conditions like eczema or dermatitis. While chamomile's efficacy as a soothing agent is well-documented, it is essential to note that it can also cause allergic reactions in individuals sensitive to ragweed or similar plants. Therefore, patch testing is recommended for new users to ensure compatibility.

Witch hazel, derived from the leaves and bark of the Hamamelis virginiana plant, is frequently marketed as a natural toner and astringent. It contains tannins, which are thought to tighten the skin and reduce inflammation. While witch hazel can help reduce oiliness and minimize the appearance of pores, its alcohol content can be drying and irritating, particularly for those with sensitive or dry skin. The effectiveness of witch hazel largely depends on its formulation; products with high alcohol content may cause more harm than good, stripping the skin of its natural oils and leading to increased sensitivity.

Rosehip oil has gained popularity for its nourishing and anti-aging properties. Rich in essential fatty acids, vitamins A and C, and antioxidants, rosehip oil is known for its ability to hydrate the skin, improve elasticity, and reduce the appearance of scars and hyperpigmentation. It is particularly beneficial for dry and mature skin, helping to strengthen the skin barrier and promote a more even skin tone. Scientific studies have shown that rosehip oil can enhance skin regeneration and improve overall skin texture, confirming its status as a valuable natural ingredient.

On the other hand, some natural ingredients are more hype than help, often included in formulations for their marketing appeal rather than their proven efficacy. **Coconut oil**, for example, is widely promoted for its moisturizing properties. While coconut oil is effective at sealing in moisture for dry skin, it is highly comedogenic, meaning it can clog pores and exacerbate acne in oily or acne-prone skin types. The molecular size of coconut oil also makes it more likely to sit on top of the skin rather than penetrate deeply, limiting its moisturizing benefits to the surface layer. For those with acne-prone skin, non-comedogenic oils like jojoba or squalane may be better alternatives.

Essential oils, such as lavender, tea tree, and peppermint, are often marketed for their natural antibacterial and anti-inflammatory properties. While there is some evidence supporting the efficacy of certain essential oils in treating acne or calming the skin, their high concentration can lead to irritation, allergic reactions, or sensitization, especially with prolonged use. Tea tree oil, for instance, has been shown to have antimicrobial properties, but it must be diluted properly to avoid skin irritation. Essential oils should be used with caution, and individuals with sensitive skin should consider avoiding them altogether or opting for products specifically formulated with safe concentrations.

Charcoal is another ingredient that has garnered attention for its supposed detoxifying benefits. While activated charcoal can absorb impurities and excess oil from the skin, there is limited scientific evidence to support its effectiveness as a skincare ingredient. Charcoal masks and cleansers may provide temporary benefits for oily skin by drawing out dirt and oil from the pores, but they can also be drying and may cause irritation with frequent use. The benefits of charcoal in skincare are largely anecdotal, and its popularity is often driven by marketing trends rather than robust scientific validation.

The use of **apple cider vinegar** in skincare is a trend that has gained traction due to its natural origins and purported benefits for balancing the skin's pH and treating acne. However, apple cider vinegar is highly acidic and can cause burns, irritation, and damage to the skin barrier if not properly diluted. There is limited scientific evidence to support its use in skincare, and its risks often outweigh the potential benefits. Professional-grade acids, such as glycolic or salicylic acid, are more effective and safer alternatives for exfoliation and acne treatment.

When evaluating natural ingredients in skincare, it is important to rely on scientific evidence and consider the ingredient's formulation, concentration, and potential for irritation. Just because an ingredient is natural does not automatically make it safe or effective for all skin types. Patch testing, consulting with a dermatologist, and focusing on evidence-based skincare are crucial steps in choosing products that genuinely benefit the skin rather than falling victim to marketing claims. Understanding the true potential and limitations of natural ingredients can help individuals make more informed choices and achieve healthier, more balanced skin.

6.3 Marketing in Skincare: What's Behind the Claims

The skincare industry is a multibillion-dollar market, driven by a powerful blend of science, innovation, and marketing. While many skincare brands genuinely aim to deliver effective products, marketing strategies often play a significant role in shaping consumer perceptions and influencing purchasing decisions. Understanding the tactics used in skincare marketing, and learning how to distinguish between truthful and misleading claims, is essential for making informed choices and avoiding the pitfalls of hype and misinformation.

One common marketing strategy is the use of **buzzwords** such as "natural," "organic," "clean," "non-toxic," and "chemical-free." These terms are designed to appeal to consumers seeking safer, more environmentally friendly options. However, these labels can be misleading, as there is no universal regulation or standard that defines what these terms mean in the context of skincare. For example, a product labeled "natural" may still contain synthetic preservatives or irritants, while "chemical-free" is a misnomer, as all substances, natural or synthetic, are composed of chemicals. The key is to look beyond these buzzwords and examine the ingredient list and scientific evidence supporting a product's claims.

Another prevalent marketing tactic is the promotion of **miracle ingredients** or **hero ingredients** that are claimed to be the solution for all skin concerns. Ingredients like hyaluronic acid, retinol, vitamin C, and peptides often receive significant attention for their scientifically proven benefits. While these ingredients can be highly effective, the concentration, formulation, and delivery method in the product are crucial factors that determine their efficacy. A product boasting a "miracle ingredient" may not provide the desired results if the ingredient is present in insufficient amounts or is not formulated correctly to penetrate the skin effectively. Consumers should seek out products with clearly stated concentrations of active ingredients and look for clinical studies or dermatologist endorsements to support the claims.

Skincare marketing also frequently employs **before-and-after photos** and **testimonials** to demonstrate a product's effectiveness. While these can be persuasive, they are often selectively chosen and do not necessarily represent the average results. Before-and-after photos can be manipulated through lighting, makeup, or digital enhancements to exaggerate the outcomes. Testimonials, while genuine in some cases, may also be biased or influenced by financial incentives or free product offers. Consumers should critically assess these images and reviews and consider whether they come from credible, independent sources or if they are featured on the brand's own marketing materials.

Another misleading practice involves the use of **clinical-sounding terms and claims** to create a sense of scientific credibility. Phrases like "clinically proven," "dermatologist-tested," and "patented formula" suggest that a product has undergone rigorous testing and has scientific backing. However, these terms are not always regulated, and the details of these studies are often not disclosed. A product that is "dermatologist-tested" does not necessarily mean it is effective or suitable for all skin types; it could simply mean a dermatologist was involved in some capacity during development. Similarly, a "patented formula" only means that the formulation is unique, not necessarily that it is effective. To verify the legitimacy of these claims, consumers should look for peer-reviewed studies published in reputable scientific journals or seek recommendations from trusted skincare professionals.

The concept of **"anti-aging"** is another area where marketing can be misleading. Many products claim to "reverse aging" or "eliminate wrinkles," playing on the fears and insecurities associated with aging. However, while skincare can significantly improve the appearance of the skin and delay the signs of aging, it cannot stop the natural aging process altogether. Effective anti-aging products typically focus on hydration, sun protection, and active ingredients like retinoids, antioxidants, and peptides that can help reduce the appearance of fine lines and improve skin texture. It is important to set realistic expectations and understand that skincare is about maintenance and gradual improvement rather than immediate, miraculous results.

The rise of **influencer marketing** has also significantly impacted the skincare industry. Influencers often promote skincare products on social media platforms, sharing their personal experiences and results. While some influencers provide valuable insights and honest reviews, others may promote products primarily for financial gain or due to brand partnerships. Consumers should be aware that influencers may not always have the expertise or qualifications to provide reliable skincare advice. It is beneficial to seek information from dermatologists, licensed estheticians, or scientific resources rather than relying solely on influencer recommendations.

In addition to these tactics, the concept of **"clean beauty"** has gained traction, with brands emphasizing the exclusion of certain ingredients deemed harmful or controversial, such as parabens, sulfates, and phthalates. While this approach appeals to consumers looking for safer products, it is important to note that the safety of these ingredients is often context-dependent, and their exclusion does not automatically make a product superior. Many excluded ingredients are used in very low concentrations, deemed safe by regulatory bodies, and are effective in preserving product stability and preventing bacterial growth. Consumers should focus on evidence-based formulations and understand that "free-from" claims are not always indicative of a product's quality or safety.

To navigate the complexities of skincare marketing and make informed decisions, consumers should adopt a skeptical and discerning approach:

- **Read Ingredient Lists**: Understanding the ingredients in a product is crucial. Look for evidence-based ingredients that are known to be effective for your specific skin concerns. Pay attention to the order of ingredients, as they are listed by concentration. Active ingredients should be among the top listed for maximum efficacy.

- **Seek Credible Sources**: Research products through reputable sources, such as dermatologists, licensed skincare professionals, or peer-reviewed scientific literature. Websites, blogs, and forums that provide unbiased, evidence-based reviews can also be valuable resources.

- **Question Claims**: Be cautious of products that promise instant or miraculous results. Effective skincare often requires consistency and time. Question vague claims like "clinically proven" without supporting evidence and be wary of products that rely heavily on testimonials and before-and-after photos.

- **Understand Your Skin Type and Concerns**: Skincare is highly individual, and what works for one person may not work for another. Understanding your skin type and concerns can help you choose products that are genuinely beneficial rather than those marketed to a broad audience.

By recognizing the strategies used in skincare marketing and critically evaluating product claims, consumers can make more informed choices, invest in truly effective skincare, and avoid falling victim to misleading marketing tactics.

BONUS – DIY FACE MASKS

1. Introduction to DIY Face Masks

DIY face masks have become increasingly popular as people seek more natural and personalized skincare solutions. The appeal of creating your own skincare treatments at home lies not only in the control over the ingredients used but also in the ability to tailor these treatments to specific skin needs. By using fresh, natural ingredients, you can ensure that your skin is receiving pure and potent nutrients without the potential irritants and chemicals found in many commercial skincare products.

One of the key benefits of DIY face masks is their ability to be customized to your skin type and concerns. Whether you have dry, oily, combination, or sensitive skin, you can select ingredients that address your specific needs. For instance, ingredients like honey and avocado provide deep hydration for dry skin, while ingredients like green clay and lemon are perfect for controlling excess oil and balancing oily skin. This level of customization is rarely achievable with store-bought products, which are often formulated for a broad audience and may not address your unique skincare challenges.

The use of fresh ingredients in DIY face masks also ensures that your skin benefits from the highest potency of active compounds. Ingredients like fruits, vegetables, and herbs contain vitamins, antioxidants, and enzymes that degrade over time. By preparing masks fresh, right before application, you maximize the efficacy of these natural compounds. For example, freshly prepared masks with ingredients like papaya, which is rich in enzymes, or strawberries, which are high in vitamin C, can help exfoliate and brighten the skin more effectively than products that have been sitting on a shelf for months.

Another advantage of DIY face masks is the reduction of exposure to potentially harmful additives found in commercial skincare products. Many mass-produced face masks contain preservatives, artificial fragrances, and colors that can cause irritation, especially for those with sensitive skin. By making your own masks, you can avoid these ingredients entirely, reducing the risk of allergic reactions and irritation. This is particularly beneficial for individuals with specific sensitivities or allergies, who often struggle to find suitable products in the market.

DIY face masks also encourage a mindful skincare routine, allowing you to connect with the ingredients and understand their benefits more deeply. This hands-on approach fosters a greater appreciation for natural ingredients and their roles in skincare, promoting a holistic view of skin health that goes beyond just the surface. Engaging in the process of selecting, preparing, and applying these masks can be a form of self-care, providing a relaxing, spa-like experience in the comfort of your own home.

Moreover, the simplicity and affordability of DIY face masks make them accessible to everyone. With just a few ingredients commonly found in your kitchen, you can create effective skincare treatments without the need for expensive products or salon visits. This accessibility allows you to experiment with different ingredients and combinations to find what works best for your skin, all while keeping skincare costs manageable.

The trend of DIY face masks aligns with a broader movement towards clean beauty and sustainable living. By using ingredients from your pantry or garden, you reduce waste associated with packaging and support a more eco-friendly skincare routine. This approach not only benefits your skin but also contributes to a more sustainable and conscious lifestyle, aligning with the values of many modern consumers who are increasingly aware of their environmental impact.

Incorporating DIY face masks into your skincare regimen can provide a multitude of benefits, from personalized care and ingredient transparency to cost savings and environmental responsibility. With the right ingredients and a bit of creativity, you can transform simple kitchen staples into powerful skincare treatments that nourish, protect, and rejuvenate your skin naturally.

Benefits of Natural Masks

Using natural ingredients in face masks offers several distinct advantages over commercial skincare products, primarily due to their purity, potency, and the absence of potentially harmful additives. One of the most significant benefits of natural masks is the reduced risk of irritation and allergic reactions. Many commercial skincare products contain synthetic fragrances, preservatives, and other chemicals that can cause sensitivity, redness, and breakouts, especially for individuals with sensitive or reactive skin. Natural ingredients, on the other hand, are less likely to provoke these reactions, particularly when chosen carefully to match one's skin type and concerns.

Natural ingredients are often gentler on the skin compared to their synthetic counterparts. Ingredients like honey, oatmeal, and aloe vera have been used for centuries for their soothing and healing properties. They contain natural anti-inflammatory and moisturizing agents that can calm irritated skin and provide deep hydration without clogging pores or causing breakouts. This makes them ideal for sensitive skin types or for those experiencing conditions such as eczema, rosacea, or dermatitis. Additionally, natural masks can be easily customized to exclude any ingredients known to cause irritation or allergies, providing a tailored skincare solution that is difficult to find in the commercial market.

Another advantage of natural masks is their ability to deliver a concentrated dose of vitamins, minerals, and antioxidants directly to the skin. Fresh fruits, vegetables, and herbs are rich in nutrients that nourish the skin, protect against environmental damage, and promote a healthy, radiant complexion. For instance, ingredients like avocado and olive oil are high in essential fatty acids and vitamin E, which help to strengthen the skin's natural barrier and lock in moisture. Turmeric, a popular ingredient in natural masks, contains curcumin, a powerful antioxidant that fights free radicals and reduces inflammation. These natural compounds are often more effective when they are fresh and unprocessed, as they retain their full potency and bioavailability.

Natural masks also offer a level of transparency that is not always available with commercial products. When you create a mask at home, you know exactly what ingredients are being used and can avoid any unnecessary fillers, preservatives, or synthetic chemicals that may be present in store-bought masks. This transparency allows for greater control over what you are applying to your skin, ensuring that only beneficial, non-toxic ingredients are used. For individuals concerned with clean beauty or who have ethical preferences regarding ingredient sourcing and testing, natural masks provide a more straightforward and conscientious option.

In addition to their safety and efficacy, natural masks often support sustainable and eco-friendly practices. By using ingredients readily available in your kitchen or garden, you minimize packaging waste and reduce your carbon footprint. Many commercial products are packaged in single-use plastics and other materials that contribute to environmental pollution. By choosing natural, homemade masks, you contribute to a more sustainable skincare routine that aligns with broader environmental values.

Natural ingredients also allow for more flexibility and creativity in skincare. You can easily mix and match ingredients to create a mask that suits your specific needs, whether it's hydration, exfoliation, brightening, or soothing. For example, adding a few drops of tea tree oil to a clay mask can enhance its acne-fighting properties, while blending yogurt with honey can create a nourishing mask that soothes and hydrates dry skin. This level of customization ensures that each mask can be tailored to address individual skin concerns effectively.

Finally, natural masks provide a holistic approach to skincare that goes beyond mere aesthetics. The process of preparing and applying a mask can be a therapeutic and mindful experience, promoting relaxation and self-care. This ritualistic aspect of skincare can help reduce stress, which is known to exacerbate various skin conditions, including acne and eczema. By taking the time to care for your skin with natural, nourishing ingredients, you also foster a deeper connection to your body and its needs, enhancing overall well-being.

By embracing the benefits of natural masks, individuals can achieve healthier, more balanced skin while also promoting a more conscious and environmentally friendly skincare routine. This approach to skincare not only helps in maintaining a radiant complexion but also aligns with the principles of clean beauty and sustainable living.

2. General Preparation Tips

Creating an effective DIY face mask requires careful preparation to ensure that the ingredients work harmoniously with your skin, delivering maximum benefits without causing irritation or adverse reactions. Proper preparation is key to a successful at-home facial treatment, and it involves several important steps, from cleansing the skin to measuring ingredients accurately and knowing the appropriate application time. Here are some essential tips to guide you through the process of preparing a DIY face mask.

Start with a Clean Canvas

Before applying any face mask, it's crucial to begin with a thoroughly cleansed face. Cleansing removes dirt, oil, makeup, and impurities that can create a barrier between your skin and the mask, preventing the ingredients from penetrating effectively. Use a gentle cleanser suited to your skin type—gel cleansers for oily skin, cream or oil-based cleansers for dry skin, and micellar water or mild foaming cleansers for sensitive skin. After cleansing, gently pat your face dry with a soft towel. Avoid rubbing, as this can irritate the skin and cause unnecessary friction, especially if your skin is sensitive or prone to redness.

Measure Ingredients Accurately

When preparing a DIY face mask, accurate ingredient dosing is essential to achieve the desired results and prevent skin irritation. Some natural ingredients, like lemon juice or baking soda, are potent and can be irritating if used in excessive amounts. Follow the recipe measurements carefully, using standard kitchen measuring tools such as teaspoons, tablespoons, and measuring cups. If a recipe calls for a specific concentration, such as a few drops of essential oil, be precise in your measurements to ensure safety and efficacy. Overuse of potent ingredients can lead to skin sensitivity, dryness, or even chemical burns.

Mix to the Right Consistency

The texture of your mask should be smooth and easy to apply. If the mask is too thick, it may not spread evenly across your face, leading to uneven treatment. If it's too runny, it could drip and make a mess, reducing the effectiveness of the treatment. Use a clean bowl and a spoon or spatula to mix your ingredients until you achieve a creamy, paste-like consistency. Some masks may require a bit of tweaking; for example, adding a little extra yogurt or honey can help to achieve the desired texture without compromising the mask's effectiveness. If your mask includes clays or powders, add liquids slowly while stirring to avoid clumping.

Application Techniques

Using the right application technique can enhance the effectiveness of your DIY face mask. Apply the mask evenly across your face using clean fingers or a brush designed for mask application. Begin at the center of your face and work your way outward, avoiding the delicate eye and lip areas. Ensure that you cover all areas that require treatment but avoid applying the mask too close to your eyes or mouth, as these areas have thinner, more sensitive skin. Applying a thick, even layer ensures that all areas receive an adequate amount of the mask's active ingredients.

Know the Right Duration

The duration for which you leave a face mask on can significantly impact its effectiveness. Most masks should be left on for about 10 to 20 minutes, allowing enough time for the ingredients to penetrate the skin and deliver their benefits. However, this can vary depending on the ingredients used. For example, masks containing gentle ingredients like honey or oatmeal can be left on for longer, while those with stronger active ingredients, such as citrus or clay, may need to be removed sooner to prevent irritation. Set a timer to ensure you do not exceed the recommended duration, and always listen to your skin—if you experience any discomfort or irritation, rinse the mask off immediately.

Rinsing Off Properly

Proper removal of the mask is just as important as the application. Use lukewarm water to rinse off the mask gently. Hot water can strip the skin of its natural oils and cause irritation, while cold water may not effectively remove all residues. Use circular motions to gently massage the skin as you rinse, helping to enhance circulation and promote relaxation. For masks that are more stubborn to remove, such as those containing honey or oatmeal, use a soft washcloth dampened with lukewarm water to aid in the removal. Be gentle to avoid tugging at the skin, which can cause redness or irritation.

Follow Up with Skincare

After removing your DIY face mask, it's essential to follow up with appropriate skincare to lock in the benefits and further protect your skin. Start with a toner to balance your skin's pH levels, followed by a serum that addresses your specific skin concerns, such as hydration, anti-aging, or brightening. Finish with a moisturizer to seal in the hydration and keep your skin soft and supple. If you're applying the mask during the daytime, don't forget to apply a broad-spectrum sunscreen with at least SPF 30, as some ingredients can make your skin more sensitive to sunlight.

By following these preparation tips, you can maximize the effectiveness of your DIY face masks, ensuring they are both safe and beneficial for your skin. With the right approach and attention to detail, your homemade masks can provide the same level of care and results as professional treatments, bringing a touch of spa-like luxury to your home routine.

Safety Tips

When creating and using DIY face masks, safety should always be a top priority. While natural ingredients can offer numerous benefits, they can also cause allergic reactions or irritations, especially for those with sensitive skin. Performing a patch test before applying a new mask is a simple yet essential step to ensure that the ingredients are safe for your skin type. Additionally, understanding which ingredients to avoid can help prevent adverse reactions and maintain healthy, glowing skin.

How to Perform a Patch Test

A patch test helps determine whether your skin might react negatively to a new ingredient or product. To perform a patch test, follow these steps:

1. **Choose a Small Area**: Select a small, inconspicuous area of skin to test the mask, such as the inside of your wrist, behind your ear, or along the jawline. These areas are less visible and are typically sensitive enough to indicate potential reactions without affecting larger, more noticeable areas of the face.

2. **Apply a Small Amount**: Take a small amount of the prepared mask and apply it to the chosen area. Ensure that the mask covers only a small patch of skin to limit exposure in case of an adverse reaction.

3. **Wait for 24 Hours**: Leave the mask on for the recommended duration, typically 10-15 minutes, then rinse it off thoroughly with lukewarm water. Wait for 24 hours to observe how your skin reacts. Look for signs of redness, itching, swelling, or any other form of irritation. If any of these symptoms occur, it indicates that the mask or one of its ingredients may not be suitable for your skin.

4. **Check for Delayed Reactions**: Sometimes, skin reactions can be delayed. Even if your skin appears fine immediately after rinsing, monitor the area over the next 24 hours for any delayed signs of irritation or sensitivity.

5. **Proceed with Caution**: If the patch test area remains clear without any signs of irritation or discomfort, the mask is likely safe to use on your face. However, if you

notice any reaction, it is best to avoid using the mask entirely or consider modifying the recipe to exclude the triggering ingredient.

Ingredients to Avoid for Sensitive Skin Types

Sensitive skin requires extra care, and certain ingredients, even natural ones, can be too harsh or irritating. Here are some ingredients commonly found in DIY masks that those with sensitive skin may want to avoid:

- **Citrus Fruits (Lemon, Orange, Grapefruit)**: While citrus fruits are popular in DIY masks for their brightening properties, their high acidity can irritate sensitive skin, leading to redness and discomfort. The acids can also increase skin's sensitivity to the sun, raising the risk of sunburn.

- **Essential Oils**: While essential oils like tea tree, peppermint, and lavender have antimicrobial and soothing properties, they are highly concentrated and can cause irritation or allergic reactions if not properly diluted. People with sensitive skin should use essential oils with caution and always perform a patch test before full application.

- **Baking Soda**: Often used in DIY masks for its exfoliating and brightening effects, baking soda can be too alkaline for the skin's natural pH, leading to dryness, irritation, and disruption of the skin barrier. It is best avoided by those with sensitive or reactive skin.

- **Raw Apple Cider Vinegar**: Though apple cider vinegar is touted for its astringent properties and ability to balance skin pH, its high acidity can be too harsh for sensitive skin, causing burns, redness, and irritation. It should be heavily diluted if used, but even then, sensitive skin types may want to steer clear.

- **Physical Exfoliants (Sugar, Salt, Ground Nuts)**: While physical exfoliants can help remove dead skin cells, their abrasive nature can cause microtears in sensitive skin, leading to irritation and inflammation. Gentle, non-abrasive ingredients like oatmeal or finely ground rice powder are better alternatives for exfoliation in sensitive skin types.

- **Honey**: Although honey is generally soothing and beneficial, it can cause allergic reactions in some people, particularly those with allergies to pollen or bee products. It's essential to ensure you have no known allergies before using honey in DIY skincare.

General Safety Precautions

- **Use Fresh Ingredients**: Always use fresh ingredients when preparing DIY face masks to avoid bacterial contamination and ensure maximum efficacy. Stale or expired ingredients can harbor bacteria and cause infections or breakouts.

- **Avoid Prolonged Storage**: DIY masks do not contain preservatives, so it's best to prepare them fresh each time and avoid storing them for future use. If you must store a mask, keep it in a clean, airtight container in the refrigerator and use it within a day or two to minimize the risk of bacterial growth.

- **Monitor Skin's Reaction**: Pay close attention to how your skin responds not just to individual masks but also to your overall skincare routine. If you notice persistent redness, dryness, or sensitivity, it may be a sign that certain ingredients or combinations are not suitable for your skin.

By following these safety tips and being mindful of ingredient choices, you can enjoy the benefits of DIY face masks without compromising your skin's health. Taking the time to perform a patch test and avoid potentially irritating ingredients is a small investment for the long-term well-being of your skin.

3. Masks for Dry Skin

Recipe 1: Honey and Avocado Mask

List of Ingredients:

- 1/2 ripe avocado

- 1 tablespoon of raw honey

- 1 teaspoon of plain yogurt (optional for extra hydration)

Step-by-Step Procedure:

1. **Prepare the Ingredients**: Start by halving a ripe avocado and removing the pit. Scoop out half of the avocado into a small mixing bowl. Make sure the avocado is ripe to ensure it's soft and easy to mash.

2. **Mash the Avocado**: Using a fork or spoon, mash the avocado until it reaches a smooth, creamy consistency. Avocado is rich in healthy fats and vitamins that nourish and hydrate the skin.

3. **Add the Honey**: Add one tablespoon of raw honey to the mashed avocado. Honey acts as a natural humectant, meaning it draws moisture into the skin, making it ideal for combating dryness. Stir well to combine the two ingredients into a uniform paste.

4. **Include Yogurt (Optional)**: If your skin is particularly dry or you're looking for an extra boost of hydration, add a teaspoon of plain yogurt to the mixture. Yogurt

contains lactic acid, which gently exfoliates dead skin cells, allowing better absorption of the mask's nourishing ingredients. Mix until smooth.

5. **Apply the Mask**: Before applying the mask, make sure your face is clean and free from any makeup or impurities. Using clean fingers or a brush, apply the mask evenly across your face, avoiding the eye and lip areas. Ensure that the mask is spread in a thick layer for maximum benefit.

6. **Leave on for 15-20 Minutes**: Allow the mask to sit on your face for about 15 to 20 minutes. This gives the ingredients time to penetrate the skin and deliver hydration and nourishment. Use this time to relax, perhaps with a good book or some calming music.

7. **Rinse Off**: After the time is up, rinse the mask off with lukewarm water. Gently massage your skin in circular motions while rinsing to help remove any residue. Pat your face dry with a soft towel, avoiding any harsh rubbing.

8. **Follow Up with Skincare**: To seal in the moisture from the mask, apply a hydrating serum or facial oil, followed by a rich moisturizer suited for dry skin. This helps to lock in the hydration and leaves your skin feeling soft and supple.

Specific Benefits for Dry Skin:

The Honey and Avocado Mask is an excellent choice for those with dry skin due to its deeply hydrating and nourishing properties. Avocado is packed with fatty acids, such as oleic acid, which helps to moisturize and repair the skin barrier. It also contains vitamins E and C, which are antioxidants that protect the skin from environmental damage and promote healing.

Honey, on the other hand, is renowned for its humectant properties, drawing moisture from the air into the skin and helping to keep it hydrated. It also has antibacterial and anti-inflammatory properties, which can soothe dry, irritated skin and prevent breakouts that sometimes occur when the skin's barrier is compromised.

The optional addition of yogurt adds an extra layer of benefit, as it gently exfoliates with its lactic acid content, removing dead skin cells that can make dry skin appear dull and flaky. This mild exfoliation allows for better penetration of the mask's other ingredients, enhancing their moisturizing effects.

Overall, this mask provides a powerful combination of hydration, nourishment, and gentle exfoliation, making it perfect for reviving dry, lackluster skin. Regular use can help restore your skin's natural glow, improve its texture, and leave it feeling soft and deeply moisturized.

Recipe 2: Banana and Yogurt Mask

List of Ingredients:

- 1/2 ripe banana

- 2 tablespoons of plain yogurt

- 1 teaspoon of honey

Step-by-Step Procedure:

1. **Prepare the Ingredients**: Begin by peeling a ripe banana and cutting it in half. Place half of the banana into a mixing bowl. Bananas should be ripe, as they are softer and easier to mash, and their nutrient content is more bioavailable in this state.

2. **Mash the Banana**: Use a fork to mash the banana until it is smooth and free of lumps. Bananas are rich in potassium and vitamin A, which help to hydrate and nourish dry skin while promoting skin cell renewal.

3. **Add the Yogurt**: Add two tablespoons of plain yogurt to the mashed banana. Yogurt contains lactic acid, which acts as a gentle exfoliant, removing dead skin cells and allowing the skin to better absorb moisture. Stir the mixture well until the banana and yogurt are fully combined into a creamy paste.

4. **Incorporate the Honey**: Add one teaspoon of honey to the mixture. Honey is a natural humectant that helps retain moisture in the skin, making it an ideal ingredient

for dry skin. It also provides antibacterial benefits, which can help prevent any potential breakouts. Mix all the ingredients thoroughly to ensure an even consistency.

5. **Apply the Mask**: Ensure your face is clean and dry before applying the mask. Using clean fingers or a mask brush, apply the mask evenly across your face, avoiding the delicate eye and lip areas. Apply a generous layer to ensure that the skin is fully covered and can benefit from the mask's hydrating properties.

6. **Let the Mask Sit for 15-20 Minutes**: Allow the mask to sit on your skin for 15 to 20 minutes. This duration allows the ingredients to penetrate deeply into the skin, providing hydration and nourishment. During this time, try to relax and let the mask work its magic.

7. **Rinse Off**: Use lukewarm water to rinse the mask off gently. As you rinse, massage your skin in circular motions to enhance circulation and help remove the mask. Ensure all traces of the mask are removed, especially around the hairline and jawline. Pat your skin dry with a soft towel.

8. **Moisturize**: After rinsing off the mask, follow up with a hydrating toner and a rich moisturizer to lock in the hydration provided by the mask. If desired, apply a few drops of facial oil for added moisture and a dewy finish.

Specific Benefits for Dry Skin:

The Banana and Yogurt Mask is particularly beneficial for dry skin due to its combination of hydrating, nourishing, and exfoliating ingredients. Bananas are packed with potassium, a vital mineral that helps to maintain skin hydration and prevent dryness. They also contain natural oils that help to moisturize and soften the skin, making them an excellent choice for combating dryness.

Yogurt is rich in lactic acid, a mild alpha hydroxy acid (AHA) that gently exfoliates the skin, removing dead skin cells and promoting cell turnover. This gentle exfoliation allows the skin to better absorb moisture and nutrients from the mask and other skincare products. The probiotics in yogurt also help to maintain a healthy skin microbiome, which can be particularly beneficial for those with dry, sensitive skin.

Honey adds an extra layer of hydration and has natural humectant properties, which means it draws moisture from the environment into the skin, keeping it plump and hydrated. Honey's soothing properties also help to calm irritated skin and reduce redness, which is a common issue for those with dry or dehydrated skin.

Together, the ingredients in this mask work synergistically to provide deep hydration, gentle exfoliation, and nourishment, helping to restore dry, flaky skin to a smoother, more radiant state. Regular use of this mask can improve skin texture, enhance hydration levels, and promote a healthy, glowing complexion.

4. Masks for Oily Skin

Recipe 1: Green Clay and Lemon Mask

List of Ingredients:

- 2 tablespoons of green clay powder
- 1 teaspoon of fresh lemon juice
- 1 tablespoon of water or rose water (for a more soothing effect)

Step-by-Step Procedure:

1. **Prepare the Ingredients**: Begin by gathering all the ingredients. Green clay powder, also known as French green clay, is widely available in health stores or online. Fresh lemon juice should be squeezed from a lemon, ensuring it is free of seeds or pulp.

2. **Mix the Green Clay**: In a small bowl, combine the two tablespoons of green clay powder with one tablespoon of water or rose water. Rose water is an excellent choice if you want a more soothing mask, as it helps to calm and tone the skin. Mix well with a spoon or spatula until you achieve a smooth, thick paste.

3. **Add the Lemon Juice**: Gradually add one teaspoon of fresh lemon juice to the green clay mixture. Lemon juice is high in vitamin C and has natural astringent properties that help control excess oil and brighten the skin. Stir the mixture thoroughly to combine the ingredients. The mask should have a smooth consistency without any lumps.

4. **Apply the Mask**: Before applying the mask, ensure your face is clean and free from any makeup or oils. Using clean fingers or a mask brush, apply the mask evenly across your face, concentrating on areas that are particularly oily, such as the T-zone (forehead, nose, and chin). Avoid the delicate eye and lip areas, as the mask can be too drying for these sensitive areas.

5. **Leave on for 10-15 Minutes**: Allow the mask to sit on your face for about 10 to 15 minutes. Green clay works by absorbing excess oil and impurities from the skin, and lemon juice helps tighten pores and reduce shine. You may feel a tightening sensation as the mask dries—this is normal and indicates that the clay is working. However, if you experience any stinging or discomfort, rinse off the mask immediately.

6. **Rinse Off**: Use lukewarm water to gently rinse off the mask. It may help to use a soft washcloth to remove any remaining mask residue. Be sure to rinse thoroughly to

avoid leaving any clay behind, which could potentially dry out the skin. After rinsing, pat your face dry with a clean, soft towel.

7. **Tone and Moisturize**: Follow up with an alcohol-free toner to balance your skin's pH levels and remove any remaining impurities. Finish with a lightweight, oil-free moisturizer to hydrate the skin without adding extra oil. This step is crucial to maintain the skin's moisture balance after using a clarifying mask.

Specific Benefits for Oily Skin:

The Green Clay and Lemon Mask is an excellent choice for individuals with oily skin due to its oil-absorbing and pore-tightening properties. Green clay is renowned for its ability to draw out excess oil, dirt, and impurities from the pores. Its absorbent nature helps to reduce shine and control sebum production, making it ideal for those who struggle with frequent breakouts or an overly shiny complexion. Green clay also contains minerals such as magnesium, calcium, and potassium, which help nourish the skin and promote a healthy, balanced complexion.

Lemon juice, a natural astringent, helps tighten pores and reduce oiliness, contributing to a smoother and more refined skin texture. Its high vitamin C content also provides antioxidant protection, helping to combat free radical damage and promote a brighter, more even skin tone. However, because lemon juice is acidic, it is important to use it in moderation to avoid irritation, particularly for those with sensitive skin.

By combining these powerful ingredients, the Green Clay and Lemon Mask effectively targets the common challenges associated with oily skin, such as excess oil, enlarged pores, and a dull complexion. Regular use can help balance oil production, minimize breakouts, and improve the overall clarity and texture of the skin.

Recipe 2: Cucumber and Aloe Vera Mask

List of Ingredients:

- 1/2 cucumber, peeled and chopped
- 2 tablespoons of aloe vera gel
- 1 teaspoon of lemon juice (optional, for additional oil control)

Step-by-Step Procedure:

1. **Prepare the Ingredients**: Start by peeling half of a cucumber and chopping it into small pieces. Cucumber is known for its cooling and hydrating properties, making it an excellent choice for soothing and balancing oily skin. Ensure that the cucumber is fresh for maximum benefits.

2. **Blend the Cucumber**: Place the chopped cucumber into a blender or food processor and blend until it forms

a smooth puree. The cucumber should be fully liquefied to create a base for the mask. If you do not have a blender, you can grate the cucumber finely and then mash it with a fork or spoon to create a similar texture.

3. **Add the Aloe Vera Gel**: Transfer the cucumber puree to a mixing bowl and add two tablespoons of aloe vera gel. Aloe vera is known for its anti-inflammatory and moisturizing properties, which help to soothe the skin and reduce redness and irritation. Stir the mixture well until the cucumber and aloe vera are fully combined into a smooth, gel-like consistency.

4. **Incorporate Lemon Juice (Optional)**: If you wish to add an extra element of oil control, incorporate one teaspoon of freshly squeezed lemon juice into the mixture. Lemon juice has natural astringent properties that can help tighten pores and control excess oil. Mix thoroughly to ensure all ingredients are evenly distributed.

5. **Apply the Mask**: Before applying the mask, ensure your face is clean and free of makeup or impurities. Using clean fingers or a mask brush, apply the mask evenly across your face, focusing on areas that tend to be oilier, such as the forehead, nose, and chin. Avoid the delicate eye and lip areas, as the mask's ingredients may be too strong for these sensitive regions.

6. **Let the Mask Sit for 15-20 Minutes**: Allow the mask to rest on your face for about 15 to 20 minutes. The cucumber and aloe vera work together to hydrate and calm the skin, while the optional lemon juice helps to refine pores and control oil. You may feel a cool, soothing sensation from the cucumber and aloe vera, which is normal and indicates the mask is working to calm and balance your skin.

7. **Rinse Off**: Rinse the mask off gently with lukewarm water. It's helpful to use a soft washcloth to remove any remaining mask residue without irritating the skin. Be sure to thoroughly rinse all areas, particularly around the nose and hairline, to ensure no traces of the mask are left behind. Pat your skin dry with a soft, clean towel.

8. **Tone and Moisturize**: Follow up with a toner suitable for oily skin to help remove any excess residue and restore your skin's natural pH balance. Finish with a lightweight, non-comedogenic moisturizer to ensure your skin remains hydrated without becoming greasy. If desired, apply a mattifying serum to help control shine throughout the day.

Specific Benefits for Oily Skin:

The Cucumber and Aloe Vera Mask is an ideal choice for those with oily skin, thanks to its combination of cooling, hydrating, and oil-balancing properties. Cucumber is composed primarily of water and contains natural antioxidants, including vitamin C and caffeic acid, which help soothe irritation, reduce swelling, and refresh the skin. Its high water content also provides a gentle hydration boost without contributing to excess oiliness, making it perfect for oily skin types that still need moisture.

Aloe vera is a powerhouse ingredient known for its soothing and healing properties. It helps to calm irritated skin, reduce inflammation, and provide a lightweight layer of hydration that does not clog pores. This is particularly beneficial for oily skin, which requires careful balancing to prevent excess oil production without over-drying. Aloe vera also has natural antibacterial properties, which can help prevent acne breakouts that are common in oily skin types.

The optional addition of lemon juice enhances the mask's ability to control oil and refine pores. Lemon juice's astringent qualities help tighten the skin and reduce the appearance of pores, while its natural citric acid gently exfoliates, removing dead skin cells and preventing clogged pores. This combination can help improve skin texture and clarity, giving a more matte and refined appearance.

Together, these ingredients create a refreshing mask that provides hydration and balance, helping to control oil production, soothe inflammation, and maintain a healthy complexion. Regular use can help regulate sebum levels, reduce shine, and enhance overall skin clarity, making it a valuable addition to any oily skincare routine.

5. Masks for Combination Skin

Recipe 1: Honey and Oat Mask

List of Ingredients:

- 2 tablespoons of oats (preferably finely ground)
- 1 tablespoon of raw honey
- 1 tablespoon of plain yogurt or milk (optional for added moisture)

Step-by-Step Procedure:

1. **Prepare the Oats**: Begin by preparing the oats. For best results, use finely ground oats as they are easier to blend into a smooth paste and provide a gentle exfoliation. You can use a blender or food processor to grind the oats into a fine powder if you only have whole oats available.

2. **Mix the Honey with Oats**: In a small bowl, combine two tablespoons of finely ground oats with one tablespoon of raw honey. Honey is an excellent natural humectant that helps draw moisture into the skin, while oats are soothing and gentle, providing a mild exfoliation that helps balance combination skin. Stir the ingredients together until you have a uniform mixture.

3. **Add Yogurt or Milk (Optional)**: To add an extra layer of hydration and nourishment, mix in one tablespoon of plain yogurt or milk. Yogurt contains lactic acid, a gentle exfoliant that helps remove dead skin cells, and milk provides hydration and smoothness. Mix well until all ingredients are fully blended into a smooth paste. The mask should have a thick but spreadable consistency.

4. **Apply the Mask**: Before applying the mask, ensure your face is clean and dry. Using clean fingers or a mask brush, apply the mask evenly across your face, focusing on areas that are particularly dry or oily. For combination skin, it's often beneficial to apply a thicker layer on dry areas (such as the cheeks) and a thinner layer on oilier areas (such as the T-zone). Avoid the delicate eye and lip areas.

5. **Leave on for 15-20 Minutes**: Allow the mask to sit on your face for about 15 to 20 minutes. This time allows the honey and oats to nourish and hydrate the skin, while also gently exfoliating and balancing the different areas of the face. You may feel a slight tingling sensation as the mask dries, which is normal.

6. **Rinse Off**: Rinse the mask off with lukewarm water, gently massaging your skin in circular motions to enhance the exfoliating effect of the oats. This helps remove dead skin cells and impurities, leaving your skin feeling soft and refreshed. Ensure all traces of the mask

are removed, especially around the nose and hairline. Pat your face dry with a soft towel.

7. **Follow Up with Skincare**: After rinsing, apply a toner suitable for combination skin to balance your skin's pH levels. Follow up with a lightweight moisturizer that hydrates without adding excess oil, focusing more on drier areas. For oilier areas, consider using a mattifying serum or oil-control product to maintain balance throughout the day.

Specific Benefits for Combination Skin:

The Honey and Oat Mask is particularly well-suited for combination skin because it addresses both hydration needs and oil control. Combination skin often features dry areas, such as the cheeks, and oily areas, like the T-zone (forehead, nose, and chin). This mask provides a balanced approach to skincare by using ingredients that cater to both conditions.

Honey is a versatile ingredient that hydrates and soothes the skin without clogging pores, making it ideal for moisturizing dry patches while also preventing excess oil production in oily areas. Its natural antibacterial properties help keep the skin clear and prevent breakouts, a common issue in the oily parts of combination skin.

Oats are known for their soothing properties and act as a gentle exfoliant, which helps remove dead skin cells and unclog pores without stripping the skin of its natural oils. They are particularly beneficial for combination skin because they can absorb excess oil while still providing moisture, creating a balanced effect. Oats also contain anti-inflammatory compounds, which help reduce redness and irritation, making them ideal for sensitive or reactive areas of combination skin.

The optional addition of yogurt or milk further enhances the mask's ability to hydrate and smooth the skin. Yogurt's lactic acid provides a mild exfoliation, which helps brighten the skin and improve texture without causing irritation. Milk, with its soothing and hydrating properties, adds extra moisture to dry areas, helping to balance the overall complexion.

By incorporating this mask into your skincare routine, you can effectively address the unique needs of combination skin, achieving a smoother, more balanced, and healthier-looking complexion. Regular use can help maintain skin equilibrium, prevent breakouts, and keep your skin feeling soft and hydrated without excessive shine.

Recipe 2: Papaya and Yogurt Mask

List of Ingredients:

- 1/2 cup of ripe papaya, peeled and diced
- 2 tablespoons of plain yogurt
- 1 teaspoon of honey (optional for added hydration)

Step-by-Step Procedure:

1. **Prepare the Papaya**: Begin by peeling and dicing half a cup of ripe papaya. Ripe papaya is softer and easier to blend, and its enzyme content is more potent, which is beneficial for the skin. Ensure the papaya is fresh to maximize the mask's efficacy.

2. **Blend the Papaya**: Place the diced papaya in a blender or food processor and blend until it forms a smooth puree. If you do not have a blender, you can mash the papaya thoroughly with a fork until it reaches a smooth consistency. Papaya is rich in enzymes like papain, which help exfoliate dead skin cells and promote a brighter complexion.

3. **Add the Yogurt**: Transfer the papaya puree to a mixing bowl and add two tablespoons of plain yogurt. Yogurt contains lactic acid, a gentle exfoliant that helps remove dead skin cells and promotes cell turnover, which is essential for maintaining smooth, even-toned skin. Stir the mixture well until the papaya and yogurt are fully combined into a creamy paste.

4. **Incorporate Honey (Optional)**: For additional hydration and soothing benefits, add one teaspoon of honey to the mixture. Honey is a natural humectant that draws moisture into the skin, helping to maintain

hydration without making the skin oily. Mix thoroughly to ensure all ingredients are evenly distributed.

5. **Apply the Mask**: Before applying the mask, make sure your face is clean and dry. Using clean fingers or a mask brush, apply the mask evenly across your face, focusing on both dry and oily areas. The mask can be applied more thickly on dry areas to provide extra hydration. Avoid the delicate eye and lip areas to prevent irritation.

6. **Leave on for 10-15 Minutes**: Allow the mask to sit on your face for about 10 to 15 minutes. During this time, the enzymes in the papaya work to gently exfoliate the skin, while the yogurt and honey provide hydration and soothing effects. You may feel a slight tingling sensation as the mask works—this is normal, but if it becomes uncomfortable, rinse the mask off immediately.

7. **Rinse Off**: Rinse the mask off gently with lukewarm water. Use circular motions to help remove the mask and to lightly exfoliate the skin. This helps enhance circulation and ensures any dead skin cells are washed away. Be sure to remove all traces of the mask, especially around the nose and hairline, and pat your face dry with a soft towel.

8. **Follow Up with Skincare**: After rinsing off the mask, apply a toner suitable for combination skin to help balance the skin's pH levels and remove any remaining

impurities. Follow up with a moisturizer that suits combination skin—lightweight enough not to clog pores in oily areas but hydrating enough to nourish dry areas. Consider using a serum with hyaluronic acid or niacinamide to further balance the skin and maintain moisture.

Specific Benefits for Combination Skin:

The Papaya and Yogurt Mask is particularly beneficial for combination skin, thanks to its unique blend of exfoliating, hydrating, and balancing properties. Papaya is known for its natural enzymes, such as papain, which gently exfoliate dead skin cells without the need for abrasive scrubbing. This gentle exfoliation helps to unclog pores in oily areas, preventing breakouts and refining skin texture, while also promoting a brighter and more even skin tone.

Yogurt, with its lactic acid content, provides an additional layer of gentle exfoliation, enhancing the removal of dead skin cells and supporting cell turnover. This process helps to smooth out rough or flaky patches commonly found on the dry areas of combination skin. Yogurt also has soothing and moisturizing properties that help to calm the skin and reduce redness, making it an ideal ingredient for addressing both dryness and oiliness in one mask.

The optional addition of honey further enhances the mask's hydrating and soothing capabilities. Honey's natural humectant properties help draw moisture into the skin, keeping it hydrated and balanced without making it greasy. Its antibacterial properties also help to prevent acne, which is often a concern for those with combination skin prone to breakouts in the T-zone.

Overall, this mask provides a balanced approach to skincare for combination skin, addressing both oily and dry areas with targeted ingredients that hydrate, exfoliate, and balance. Regular use of the Papaya and Yogurt Mask can help maintain a smoother, more even complexion, reduce breakouts, and keep the skin looking healthy and refreshed.

6. Masks for Sensitive Skin

Recipe 1: Chamomile and Oat Mask

List of Ingredients:

- 2 tablespoons of oats (preferably finely ground)
- 1 tablespoon of chamomile tea (cooled)
- 1 tablespoon of aloe vera gel
- 1 teaspoon of honey (optional for extra soothing)

Step-by-Step Procedure:

1. **Prepare the Oats**: Begin by using finely ground oats for this mask. Finely ground oats are gentler on sensitive skin and blend more easily into a smooth paste. You can

use a blender or food processor to grind whole oats into a fine powder if needed.

2. **Brew the Chamomile Tea**: Brew a cup of chamomile tea using a chamomile tea bag or loose chamomile flowers. Allow the tea to steep for about 5 minutes, then let it cool to room temperature. Chamomile is known for its calming and anti-inflammatory properties, making it ideal for soothing sensitive skin.

3. **Mix the Oats with Chamomile Tea**: In a small mixing bowl, combine two tablespoons of finely ground oats with one tablespoon of cooled chamomile tea. Stir until the oats are fully moistened by the tea. Chamomile tea adds a soothing effect, while the oats provide a gentle exfoliation to remove dead skin cells without irritating the skin.

4. **Add Aloe Vera Gel**: Incorporate one tablespoon of aloe vera gel into the mixture. Aloe vera is renowned for its healing and soothing properties, making it a perfect ingredient for sensitive skin. It helps to calm redness, reduce inflammation, and provide a light layer of hydration. Mix well until all ingredients are fully combined into a smooth, spreadable paste.

5. **Include Honey (Optional)**: For added soothing benefits, add one teaspoon of honey to the mixture. Honey is a natural humectant that hydrates the skin while

also providing antibacterial and anti-inflammatory properties. It is especially beneficial for sensitive skin that is prone to redness or irritation. Stir the mixture thoroughly to ensure an even consistency.

6. **Apply the Mask**: Ensure your face is clean and free from any makeup or impurities before applying the mask. Using clean fingers or a mask brush, gently apply the mask evenly across your face, avoiding the eye and lip areas. Be particularly gentle when applying the mask to avoid irritating sensitive areas of the skin.

7. **Let the Mask Sit for 10-15 Minutes**: Allow the mask to sit on your face for about 10 to 15 minutes. This gives the ingredients time to soothe and hydrate the skin while also calming any redness or irritation. You should feel a soothing, cooling sensation as the mask works; if you experience any discomfort or stinging, rinse the mask off immediately.

8. **Rinse Off**: Gently rinse the mask off with lukewarm water. It's best to use a soft washcloth to help remove the mask without rubbing the skin too harshly. Be sure to rinse thoroughly to remove all traces of the mask, especially around the nose and hairline. Pat your skin dry with a soft, clean towel, being careful not to tug or pull on the skin.

9. **Follow Up with Skincare**: After removing the mask, apply a calming toner or facial mist suitable for sensitive skin to further soothe and hydrate. Follow with a lightweight, fragrance-free moisturizer designed for sensitive skin to lock in moisture and protect the skin barrier. Consider using a serum with ingredients like niacinamide or ceramides to strengthen the skin's natural defense mechanisms.

Specific Benefits for Sensitive Skin:

The Chamomile and Oat Mask is particularly beneficial for sensitive skin because it is formulated with ingredients known for their gentle, soothing, and anti-inflammatory properties. Oats are a well-known ingredient for calming sensitive skin due to their high content of beta-glucan, which helps to reduce redness, irritation, and itching. They also provide a gentle exfoliation that helps remove dead skin cells without causing micro-tears or irritation, which is crucial for sensitive skin types.

Chamomile is another star ingredient for sensitive skin, known for its calming effects and ability to reduce inflammation. It contains powerful antioxidants such as apigenin, which help protect the skin from environmental damage while soothing and calming irritation. The chamomile tea in this mask acts as a natural anti-inflammatory agent, helping to calm and comfort the skin.

Aloe vera gel adds a layer of hydration and soothing relief to the mask. It is widely recognized for its ability to reduce inflammation and provide a cooling sensation, which can help to calm and protect sensitive skin. Aloe vera also promotes healing and helps to strengthen the skin's barrier, making it more resilient against external irritants.

The optional addition of honey enhances the mask's soothing and moisturizing properties. Honey is a natural humectant that draws moisture into the skin, providing hydration without clogging pores or causing breakouts. Its antibacterial and anti-inflammatory properties also help to calm irritated skin, making it a gentle yet effective ingredient for sensitive skin types.

This combination of ingredients creates a mask that is both soothing and protective, making it ideal for those with sensitive skin who need to calm irritation and strengthen the skin barrier. Regular use can help reduce redness, soothe inflammation, and improve overall skin resilience, leading to a healthier, more balanced complexion.

Recipe 2: Rose and Honey Mask

List of Ingredients:

- 1 tablespoon of rose petal powder (or finely ground dried rose petals)

- 1 tablespoon of raw honey

- 1 teaspoon of rose water

- 1 teaspoon of aloe vera gel (optional for added soothing benefits)

Step-by-Step Procedure:

1. **Prepare the Rose Petal Powder**: If you are using dried rose petals, start by grinding them into a fine powder using a spice grinder or food processor. Alternatively, you can purchase pre-made rose petal powder from a natural health store. Rose petals are known for their calming properties and their ability to help soothe and hydrate sensitive skin.

2. **Combine the Rose Petal Powder and Honey**: In a small mixing bowl, combine one tablespoon of rose petal powder with one tablespoon of raw honey. Honey is an excellent natural humectant that helps retain moisture in the skin while also providing antibacterial and anti-inflammatory properties. Stir the ingredients together until a smooth, paste-like consistency is achieved.

3. **Add Rose Water**: Incorporate one teaspoon of rose water into the mixture. Rose water is renowned for its soothing and hydrating effects on the skin, helping to calm redness and irritation. It also adds a pleasant, natural fragrance to the mask. Mix thoroughly to combine all ingredients into a smooth, uniform paste.

4. **Include Aloe Vera Gel (Optional)**: For additional soothing benefits, add one teaspoon of aloe vera gel to the mixture. Aloe vera is known for its ability to reduce inflammation and provide a cooling effect, making it particularly beneficial for sensitive skin. Stir well to ensure all ingredients are fully blended into a smooth consistency.

5. **Apply the Mask**: Before applying the mask, ensure your face is clean and dry. Using clean fingers or a mask brush, gently apply the mask evenly across your face, avoiding the delicate eye and lip areas. Apply the mask in a thin, even layer to maximize its soothing and hydrating effects on sensitive skin.

6. **Let the Mask Sit for 10-15 Minutes**: Allow the mask to sit on your face for about 10 to 15 minutes. During this time, the rose petals, honey, and rose water work together to soothe and hydrate the skin while also calming any redness or irritation. You should feel a gentle, soothing sensation as the mask works; if you

experience any discomfort or stinging, rinse the mask off immediately.

7. **Rinse Off**: Rinse the mask off gently with lukewarm water. Use a soft washcloth to help remove any remaining mask residue without rubbing the skin too harshly. Be sure to rinse thoroughly to remove all traces of the mask, especially around the nose and hairline. Pat your skin dry with a soft, clean towel, being careful not to tug or pull on the skin.

8. **Follow Up with Skincare**: After removing the mask, apply a calming toner or facial mist designed for sensitive skin to help soothe and hydrate. Follow with a lightweight, fragrance-free moisturizer to lock in moisture and protect the skin barrier. Consider using a serum with soothing ingredients like niacinamide or allantoin to further calm the skin and enhance its resilience against environmental stressors.

Specific Benefits for Sensitive Skin:

The Rose and Honey Mask is particularly beneficial for sensitive skin due to its gentle, soothing, and hydrating properties. Rose petals and rose water are known for their calming effects on the skin. They help to reduce redness, soothe irritation, and provide a light layer of hydration, making them ideal for sensitive skin types that are prone to inflammation and sensitivity.

Honey adds another layer of benefits to this mask by acting as a natural humectant, drawing moisture into the skin to keep it hydrated and supple. Its antibacterial and anti-inflammatory properties help to soothe irritated skin and prevent potential breakouts, which can sometimes occur with sensitive skin due to its compromised barrier function.

The optional addition of aloe vera gel further enhances the mask's soothing and calming properties. Aloe vera is well-known for its ability to reduce redness and inflammation, providing a cooling effect that helps to calm and protect sensitive skin. It also aids in healing and strengthening the skin barrier, making the skin more resilient against external irritants.

Together, these ingredients create a mask that provides a balanced combination of hydration, soothing, and protection, making it perfect for those with sensitive skin. Regular use can help calm irritation, reduce redness, and enhance overall skin resilience, leading to a more comfortable, healthy-looking complexion.

7. Conclusion and Final Tips

Tips on Using Masks

Incorporating DIY face masks into your skincare routine can provide numerous benefits, from hydration and exfoliation to soothing and balancing the skin. However, to maximize their effectiveness and ensure they are safe for regular use, it's essential to follow some best practices regarding how often to use them, how to store any leftovers, and how to integrate different masks into your beauty routine.

How Often to Use Masks

The frequency with which you use face masks depends largely on your skin type and the specific needs of your skin. For most people, applying a face mask once or twice a week is sufficient to provide additional care without overloading the skin. However, different masks serve different purposes:

- **Hydrating Masks**: These can be used more frequently, especially if your skin is dry or dehydrated. Masks with ingredients like honey, avocado, or yogurt provide intense hydration and can be applied two to three times a week, depending on your skin's needs.

- **Exfoliating Masks**: Masks that contain exfoliating ingredients, such as papaya, yogurt, or oats, should be used less frequently, around once a week. Over-exfoliation can lead to irritation, redness, and a weakened skin barrier, particularly for sensitive skin types.

- **Purifying Masks**: Masks designed to draw out impurities and reduce excess oil, such as those containing green clay or lemon, should also be used once a week. For oily or acne-prone skin, you may use these masks up to twice a week, but be careful to monitor your skin's reaction to avoid over-drying.

- **Soothing Masks**: For sensitive or irritated skin, soothing masks containing ingredients like chamomile, aloe vera, or rose water can be used as often as needed, depending on the level of irritation. These masks provide gentle care and can help calm and nourish the skin after a day in harsh weather or following an irritating skincare treatment.

How to Store Leftovers

DIY face masks are best used fresh to ensure the maximum potency of their natural ingredients. However, if you have leftover mask mixture, here are some guidelines on how to store it safely:

- **Refrigerate Immediately**: Any leftover mask should be stored in an airtight container and placed in the refrigerator immediately. The cool temperature will help preserve the ingredients and prevent bacterial growth.

Most DIY masks can be kept in the fridge for up to 24 to 48 hours. Beyond this period, the mask may lose its efficacy and could potentially become unsafe to use.

- **Avoid Contamination**: Always use clean utensils and containers when preparing and storing your masks. Avoid dipping your fingers directly into the container to prevent introducing bacteria. Use a clean spoon or spatula to scoop out the desired amount for each use.

- **Check for Freshness**: Before reusing a stored mask, check for any signs of spoilage, such as changes in color, texture, or smell. If the mask appears different from when it was first prepared, it's best to discard it and make a fresh batch to ensure your skin's safety.

Integrating Different Masks into Your Routine

To get the most out of your DIY face masks, consider how to integrate them into your overall skincare routine:

- **Target Different Concerns with Multi-Masking**: If you have combination skin or specific areas that require different treatments, consider multi-masking. This involves applying different masks to different areas of your face at the same time—for example, a hydrating mask on the cheeks and a purifying mask on the T-zone. Multi-masking allows you to address multiple skin concerns in a single session.

- **Follow Up with Skincare Products**: After rinsing off a mask, it's essential to follow up with appropriate skincare products. Always start with a toner to balance your skin's pH, followed by serums that target your specific concerns (hydration, anti-aging, brightening, etc.), and end with a moisturizer to lock in all the benefits. If you've used an exfoliating or purifying mask, consider using a soothing serum or cream to calm the skin.

- **Listen to Your Skin**: Pay attention to how your skin responds to each mask and adjust your routine accordingly. If you notice any signs of irritation or discomfort, reduce the frequency of use or switch to a different mask that better suits your skin's needs. Every skin type is unique, and finding the right balance may require some experimentation.

- **Seasonal Adjustments**: Adjust your mask routine based on seasonal changes. In the winter, when the air is drier, you may need more hydrating masks. In the summer, when your skin is likely to produce more oil, purifying and balancing masks may be more beneficial.

By following these tips, you can enhance the benefits of your DIY face masks and maintain a balanced, healthy skincare routine. Regularly using masks tailored to your skin type and concerns can help achieve a more radiant, healthy complexion and provide a relaxing, spa-like experience at home.

Personalized Recommendations

Choosing the right DIY face mask involves understanding your skin's unique needs, which can vary depending on factors such as seasonality, hormonal changes, and environmental conditions. By tailoring your mask selection to these variables, you can better address specific skin concerns and maintain a balanced, healthy complexion year-round. Here are some personalized recommendations for selecting the most suitable mask based on various skin conditions:

1. Adapting to Seasonal Changes

Seasonal changes can significantly impact your skin's condition, requiring adjustments to your skincare routine:

- **Winter Months**: During the colder months, the air is typically drier, which can lead to dehydrated and flaky skin. In winter, it's essential to focus on hydrating and nourishing masks that help maintain moisture levels and protect the skin barrier. Masks with ingredients like honey, avocado, yogurt, and oatmeal are excellent choices for providing deep hydration and soothing any dryness or irritation caused by cold weather.

- **Summer Months**: In the summer, increased humidity and exposure to heat can lead to excess oil production, clogged pores, and breakouts. For summer skincare, opt for masks that help control oil and reduce shine, such as those containing green clay, cucumber, lemon juice, or aloe vera. These ingredients are effective at absorbing excess oil, tightening pores, and providing a refreshing, cooling effect on the skin.

- **Transitional Seasons (Spring and Fall)**: During transitional seasons, the skin may fluctuate between dryness and oiliness due to changes in weather and humidity. Combination skin types may benefit from multi-masking during these times, using a hydrating mask on dry areas and a purifying or balancing mask on oilier areas. Consider masks with ingredients like honey and oats for balanced hydration and green clay or papaya for oil control and gentle exfoliation.

2. Addressing Hormonal Changes

Hormonal fluctuations, such as those experienced during puberty, menstruation, pregnancy, or menopause, can significantly impact the skin:

- **Hormonal Acne**: Hormonal changes can often trigger breakouts, particularly around the chin and jawline. To address hormonal acne, choose masks with soothing and antibacterial properties to calm inflammation and prevent breakouts. Masks with ingredients like honey, tea tree oil (in small, diluted amounts), green clay, or turmeric are beneficial for acne-prone skin. These ingredients help to reduce bacteria, control oil, and soothe irritated skin without over-drying.

- **Pregnancy-Related Skin Sensitivities**: Pregnancy can cause heightened skin sensitivity, leading to redness, dryness, or even acne. During pregnancy, it's crucial to use masks that are gentle, hydrating, and free from harsh chemicals. Masks containing calming ingredients like chamomile, aloe vera, rose petals, and honey are safe and effective for soothing and nourishing sensitive skin. Always consult with a healthcare provider before trying new skincare products during pregnancy.

- **Menopause and Aging Skin**: As hormonal levels shift during menopause, skin may become drier and lose elasticity, leading to more pronounced fine lines and wrinkles. For mature skin, opt for masks that provide intense hydration and support collagen production. Ingredients such as avocado, honey, yogurt, and papaya are excellent for hydrating, firming, and brightening aging skin. These ingredients help to lock in moisture, promote cell renewal, and improve overall skin texture and tone.

3. Managing Specific Skin Conditions

In addition to seasonal and hormonal changes, other specific skin conditions may require targeted mask treatments:

- **Sensitive Skin**: Sensitive skin can react to environmental factors, harsh ingredients, or stress. To manage sensitivity, use masks formulated with soothing, calming ingredients like chamomile, oats, rose water, and aloe vera. These ingredients help to reduce inflammation, soothe irritation, and strengthen the skin's barrier without causing further sensitivity.

- **Hyperpigmentation and Dark Spots**: If you're dealing with hyperpigmentation or uneven skin tone, masks containing brightening ingredients like lemon juice (used sparingly), papaya, and yogurt can help. These ingredients offer gentle exfoliation and promote cell turnover, helping to fade dark spots over time and achieve a more even complexion. Be sure to follow up with sunscreen, as these ingredients can increase photosensitivity.

- **Rosacea and Redness**: For skin conditions like rosacea, which causes persistent redness and sensitivity, it's crucial to use ultra-soothing, anti-inflammatory masks. Ingredients like chamomile, cucumber, oats, and aloe vera are ideal for calming redness and irritation associated with rosacea. Avoid masks with strong exfoliants or acids that could exacerbate redness and irritation.

4. Customizing Based on Lifestyle and Environment

Your lifestyle and environmental exposure can also affect your skin's condition and influence your choice of face masks:

- **Urban Living and Pollution Exposure**: If you live in an urban area with high pollution levels, your skin may be more prone to oxidative stress and clogged pores. Consider detoxifying masks with ingredients like green clay, activated charcoal, or turmeric to draw out impurities, absorb excess oil, and protect against environmental damage.

- **Active Lifestyle and Frequent Sweating**: If you exercise frequently or sweat a lot, your skin may require more frequent cleansing and purifying treatments. Masks with cooling and purifying ingredients like cucumber, aloe vera, and green clay can help refresh the skin, remove impurities, and maintain a clear complexion.

By understanding how various factors such as seasonality, hormonal changes, and environmental conditions impact your skin, you can select the most suitable DIY face masks to address your specific needs. Tailoring your skincare routine to these changes will help you maintain a balanced, healthy, and radiant complexion throughout the year.

Thank you for choosing this journey to radiant, healthy skin with us. Your trust and commitment to nurturing your skin are truly appreciated. If you found value in this book, we'd love to hear your thoughts. Please consider leaving a review on Amazon—it not only helps us, but it also helps others discover the benefits of natural, effective skincare. Your feedback means the world to us!

Made in United States
North Haven, CT
13 August 2025